Social Indicators Research Series

Volume 68

This series aims to provide a public forum for single treatises and collections of papers on social indicators research that are too long to be published in our journal *Social Indicators Research*. Like the journal, the book series deals with statistical assessments of the quality of life from a broad perspective. It welcomes the research on a wide variety of substantive areas, including health, crime, housing, education, family life, leisure activities, transportation, mobility, economics, work, religion and environmental issues. These areas of research will focus on the impact of key issues such as health on the overall quality of life and vice versa. An international review board, consisting of Ruut Veenhoven, Joachim Vogel, Ed Diener, Torbjorn Moum, Mirjam A.G. Sprangers and Wolfgang Glatzer, will ensure the high quality of the series as a whole.

More information about this series at http://www.springer.com/series/6548

Tineke de Jonge • Ruut Veenhoven
Wim Kalmijn

Diversity in Survey Questions on the Same Topic

Techniques for Improving Comparability

Springer

Tineke de Jonge
Erasmus Happiness Economics Research Organisation
Erasmus University Rotterdam
Rotterdam, The Netherlands

Ruut Veenhoven
Erasmus Happiness Economics Research Organisation
Erasmus University Rotterdam
Rotterdam, The Netherlands

Wim Kalmijn (deceased)
Erasmus Happiness Economics Research Organisation
Erasmus University Rotterdam
Rotterdam, The Netherlands

ISSN 1387-6570 ISSN 2215-0099 (electronic)
Social Indicators Research Series
ISBN 978-3-319-53260-8 ISBN 978-3-319-53261-5 (eBook)
DOI 10.1007/978-3-319-53261-5

Library of Congress Control Number: 2017933832

Printed on acid-free paper

This Springer imprint is published by Springer Nature
The registered company is Springer International Publishing AG
The registered company address is: Gewerbestrasse 11, 6330 Cham, Switzerland

Preface

Today, we are investing more in scientific research than ever before in human history, and a search in Google Scholar suggests that in 2015 some eight million scientific publications were produced. All this research is assumed to result in the 'accumulation of knowledge', thought to take place through an exchange of information in this 'academic forum'. Reality is more complicated than this. There is not one academic forum, but rather many different market places, and exchange of knowledge in these bazaars is considerably hindered by the different languages and currencies used. As a result, much of the gathered information gets lost in the dust of libraries. Obstacles to accumulation of knowledge differ across academic settings. In this book, we address one particular problem in one particular research field.

This book is about a problem in survey research: in this case, large-scale questionnaire studies among samples of the general population in countries. We focus on 'social surveys' that are about the quality of life in nations. Most modern countries conduct such surveys periodically, for example, the 'Understanding Society' study in the UK, the Level of Living survey in Sweden and the Public Opinion Survey on the Life of the Nation in Japan. Then, there are international survey programs, such as the Eurobarometer, the European Social Survey, the Gallup World Poll and the World Values Survey. Worldwide, some million people take part in such surveys every year.

Social surveys address similar themes, such as social position and opinions. Many of the topics are identical; all the surveys have questions about age, sex and education, and most also ask about income and ethnicity. Yet, the questions asked on these matters are often formulated differently, for example, questions about the education level of the respondent sometimes ask the respondent to give a number for years of education, while in other surveys, a list of education types is given, from which the respondent must select the final type achieved. In this case, many different classifications of school level can be used which vary within and between countries. In this mixture of ways of asking the same question of education levels across nations and time, typically less than half of the available survey data can be used for such purpose.

One of the common topics in social surveys is ‘happiness’, that is, the satisfaction with one’s life as a whole. This matter is typically measured using single direct questions, such as: ‘Taking all together, how happy would you say you are these days? Would you say you are very happy, pretty happy or not too happy?’ To date (2016), such questions have figured in some 10,000 survey studies and have been answered by some 200,000 respondents. The observed distributions of these responses are gathered in the collection ‘Happiness in Nations’ in the World Database of Happiness (WDH) (Veenhoven 2016). Viewing this collection of data, we can see that differently formulated questions have been used and that there are also many differences in the response options presented to respondents. Again, this means that only part of the data is available for comparing happiness across nations and time. These problems are not confined to comparing levels of education and happiness across populations and nations. They are found for many other topics in survey research, such as health care or customer satisfaction,

In this book, we present methods for dealing with this diversity in survey questions on the same subject; we review existing methods used to homogenize data and propose new ones. The book is a spin-off from the World Database of Happiness, the main aim of which is to collate and make available research findings on the subjective enjoyment of life and to prepare these data for research synthesis. The first methods we discuss were proposed in the book *Happiness in Nations* (Veenhoven 1993, Chap. 7 ‘How the Data Are Homogenized’) which were used at the inception of the World Database of Happiness. Some 10 years later, a new method was introduced: the International Happiness Scale Interval Study (HSIS) (Veenhoven 2008). Taking the HSIS as a basis, Wim Kalmijn (2010) developed the Continuum Approach. Then, building on Kalmijn’s work, Tineke DeJonge (2015) developed the Reference Distribution Method.

In this book, we describe the evolution of these innovations and provide a view of where we stand now. We go on to suggest ways to evolve this line of research. The book is based on the doctoral dissertation of Tineke DeJonge (2015); most chapters are based on articles authored in most cases by the three of us and Lidia Arends of the Erasmus University Rotterdam.

Wim Kalmijn passed away in November 2015 aged 81; he contributed much to the preparation of this book. We thank Willem Saris of the University Pompeu Fabra in Barcelona for his comments on the draft version and Miranda Aldham-Breary, senior volunteer of the WDH, for improving the English.

Rotterdam, The Netherlands Ruut Veenhoven

References

De Jonge, T. (2015). *Different survey questions on the same topic. How to make responses comparable?* Dissertation, Erasmus University Rotterdam, The Netherlands. Enschede: Ipskamp Drukkers. Available at http://repub.eur.nl/pub/78339

Kalmijn, W.M. (2010). *Quantification of happiness inequality*. Dissertation, Erasmus University Rotterdam, The Netherlands. Enschede: Ipskamp Drukkers. Available at http://repub.eur.nl/pub/21777

Veenhoven, R. (1993). *Happiness in nations, subjective appreciation of life in 56 nations, 1946–1992* (Studies in social-cultural transformation, 2). Risbo, Erasmus University Rotterdam, Netherlands. Available at: https://personal.eur.nl/veenhoven/Pub1990s/93b-con.html

Veenhoven, R. (2008). The International Scale Interval Study. In V. Møller & D. Huschka (Eds.), *Quality of Life in the new millennium: 'Advances in quality-of-life studies, theory and research', Part 2: Refining concepts and measurement to assess cross-cultural quality-of-life* (Social Indicator Research Series, Vol. 35, pp. 45–58). Dordrecht: Springer Press.

Veenhoven, R. (2016). *Happiness in nations*. World Database of Happiness, Erasmus University Rotterdam. Available at: http://worlddatabaseofhappiness.eur.nl/hap_nat/nat_fp.php?mode=1

Contents

Abbreviations

BRFSS	Behavioral Risk Factor Surveillance System
CAPI	Computer-assisted personal interviewing
CBS	Statistics Netherlands
DHS	Dutch Household Survey
EAVS	East Asia Value Survey
EB	Eurobarometer
EDAC	European Data Center for Work and Welfare
EQLS	European Quality of Life Survey
ESS	European Social Survey
FLS	Future Life Survey
HSIS	Happiness Scale Interval Study
ISSP	International Periodical Social Survey Program
LAPOP	Latin American Public Opinion Project
LDC	Leisure Development Centre
LIN	Life-in-Nation Survey
LPS	Lifestyle Preference Survey
NIPO	Dutch Institute for Public Opinion
OECD	Organization for Economic Co-operation and Development
%SM	Percentage of scale maximum
SCP	The Netherlands Institute for Social Research
SWB	Subjective well-being
TRAPD	Translation, Review, Adjudication, Pretesting and Documentation
VAS	Visual analogue scale
WDH	World Database of Happiness
WVS	World Values Survey

Part I
Comparing Responses to Different Survey Questions on the Same Topic: Problems and Conventional Solutions

Chapter 1
Diversity in Survey Items and the Comparability Problem

Introduction

Survey research is a major method used in the social sciences and is largely based on standard questions with pre-coded response options called 'response scales' to which respondents answer by picking one of the options. There is little uniformity in the survey items[1] used. This difference in items is no problem when surveys are analysed separately, but it limits the comparability of findings gathered in different surveys that used different items for the same topic. This reduces the value of our accumulating of knowledge and calls for techniques to improve the comparability of data.

This diversity in the wordings of questions and in response options also appears in survey research on subjective well-being which took off in the 1970s in the wake of the Social Indicator Revolution. In this context Campbell et al. (1976) set up a program for monitoring the quality of American life, with emphasize on the experience of life rather than the, mostly material, conditions of life thus shifting the focus from current economic goals to subjective well-being. They recognized that they would encounter many problems of definitions and methods as they could not fall back on standardized measures established in earlier research which would fulfill their needs. Their main focus was upon expressions of satisfaction with specific domains of life experience, but they also included an item on happiness and an item on satisfaction with life as a whole in their survey. Andrews and Withey (1976), other pioneers in this field of research, explored a large set of survey items, among which were questions on the subjective appreciation of one's life as a whole. Many more questions designed to measure subjective well-being have been used since then. To date about a 1,000 different questions on the subjective appreciation of one's life as a whole from some 10,000 studies have been gathered in the collection 'Measures of Happiness' of the World Database of Happiness

[1]We use the term 'item' for a survey question and its corresponding response options.

T. de Jonge et al., *Diversity in Survey Questions on the Same Topic*, Social Indicators Research Series 68, DOI 10.1007/978-3-319-53261-5_1

(Veenhoven 2016a, b). About half of the differences in questions are in the number and wording of response options, other differences are due to causes such as the reference to time and the visual presentation of the scale or the method of assessment. The World Database of Happiness (WDH) focuses on happiness in the sense of the subjective enjoyment of one's life as a whole (Veenhoven 1984). In this definition 'happiness' is synonymous with 'life satisfaction'. This concept of happiness is currently the one most commonly used in the social sciences and it lies at the heart of the WDH (Veenhoven 2011).

One of the aims of happiness researchers is to assess differences in happiness across nations. This requires comparison of data drawn from different surveys containing questions about happiness. In surveys however, different kinds of response scales are used, both verbal scales and numerical scales, and these scales also differ in the number of response options available, some including only two options, for example yes or no, and others as many as 11, for example 0–10 numerical scales. As a consequence only a part of the available research can be used by scholars in any comparison or meta studies. Likewise, another aim of happiness researchers is to compare happiness within countries over time. This also requires equivalent questions and response scales, but since the response scales used can change over the years, the number of comparable data available will often be inadequate for a valid comparison to be made.

Diversity in survey items is often treated in one of two ways: one is to abstain from any comparison when rating scales are not fully identical. This means that most of the findings on happiness are incomparable and thus lost for synthetic analysis. The other approach is to ignore the problem, typically by assuming that the ranks of the response options reflect the degree of happiness denoted and treating these numbers as metric values that can be transformed to the same range. This approach carries the danger of producing nonsense.

An Impression of the Diversity in Survey Items

Most people have a positive perception of their own well-being, at least in the western world. As a result, the distribution of responses to questions on happiness is skewed, with a long tail on the left that represents 'negative' outcomes (Campbell et al. 1976; Lee et al. 1982; Diener and Diener 1996; Cummins 2003; Frijters et al. Shields 2008; Guven et al. 2011). Irrespective of the scale used, this skewness has to be kept in mind when interpreting the results of such measurements.

Within the large set of existing measures of happiness, the number of response options and the distinction between verbal and numerical response scales are obvious variations. To meet the skewness of the distribution, in the past verbal scales were devised that are asymmetric due to mainly positively formulated response options. An example of such a scale is the one used by Statistics Netherlands from 1974 to 2010, a long period, to measure satisfaction with life. Respondents were given the response options 'Extraordinarily satisfied', 'Very satisfied',

'Satisfied', 'Fairly satisfied' and 'Not very satisfied'. Note: only the latter of these responses is formulated negatively. The idea behind this rather asymmetric scale at the time it was devised was that it would give the possibility for more variation in the responses than if a more symmetric scale was used. Another, totally different example of a response scale devised to reduce the skew is provided by Andrews and Withey (1976). They argued that substantially skewed distributions pose problems in analysis and that reducing the skew in the distribution of response would therefore enhance our ability to find meaningful relationships between different aspects of life. With this in mind they felt they could improve the "satisfaction" scale used by Campbell et al. which is a symmetric numerical scale, with one anchor point[2] labeled 'Completely satisfied' and the other anchor point labeled 'Completely dissatisfied'. Andrews and Withey's improvement of this scale (1976, pp. 18–19) consisted of adding more affect to it, resulting in what is known as the Delighted-Terrible scale. This scale includes the seven on-scale options 'Delighted', 'Pleased', 'Mostly satisfied', 'Mixed – about equally satisfied and dissatisfied', 'Mostly dissatisfied', 'Unhappy' and 'Terrible', supplemented with three off-scale options 'Neutral – neither satisfied nor dissatisfied', 'Does not apply to me' and 'I never thought about it'. Andrews and Withey drawing conclusions from the numerous different ways they experimented with to measuring affect, stated they believed that this scale was the most effective.

The satisfaction with life scale used by Statistics Netherlands is a unipolar scale: all response options contain the word 'satisfied'. This differs from a bipolar scale, as for example the "Satisfaction with life scale" of Campbell et al. where in the response options, for example, the word 'dissatisfied' is used as the opponent of 'satisfied'. Furthermore, a scale does not necessarily need to have a neutral mid-point dividing it into a positive and a negative pole and the end points of different scales may vary in the extremity of the wording used, for example 'extraordinarily' is more extreme than 'very' but both are subject to a respondents interpretation of the words the effect of the context in which they are used, and this will vary from respondent to respondent.

Most of the variations discussed above hold for both verbal response scales and for numerical response scales. Although numbers are used on a numerical scale to express the respondent's degree of happiness, it is still necessary to use words to describe what the anchor points of the scale denote, and it is this wording which defines whether the scale is conceived to be unipolar or bipolar. The wording of such descriptions can include the subject of measurement, as in 'dissatisfied' – 'satisfied' or leave it to the respondents how they interpret the anchor points or extremes of the scale when a formulation is given in terms like 'best possible' – 'worst possible'. An early and well-known example of the latter is Cantril's self-anchoring Ladder of Life Scale. Using this satisfaction of life measure, respondents

[2]We use the term 'anchor points' for the response options at both ends of a discrete scale. In the case of a continuous distribution, we use the term 'extremes' to refer to the boundaries of the continuum that bounds this distribution.

are asked to imagine a ladder with steps numbered from zero at the bottom to ten at the top. The top step of the ladder represents the best possible life for the respondent and the bottom step the worst possible life. The respondents have to rate on which step of the ladder they feel they personally stand at the time of questioning. This measure was first employed for a national sample in the United States in 1959 (Campbell et al. 1976, p. 31) and is still used, for example in Gallup's World Poll (Bjørnskov 2010; Gallup 2016).

Other variations in numerical scales are the visual orientation, which can be vertical or horizontal, and the labeling of the anchor points that can go from negative to positive, for example −5 to +5, consists only of positive numbers and possibly including zero starting at 0 or 1, or there can be no numbering (Mazaheri and Theuns 2009). In an experiment done by Schwartz et al. (1991) using an 11-point numerical scale with anchor points labeled from 'Not at all successful' to 'Extremely successful' and ranging from −5 to +5 only 13% of the respondents gave an answer between −5 and 0. When the range changed from 0 to 10, the percentage of answers at the lower end of the scale changed to 34%. A similar result was found by Sangster et al. (2001). From this experiment Schwarz and his colleagues concluded that a numerical scale starting at zero suggests the absence or presence of the subject under study, which makes the scale unipolar. If conversely, one half of the scale is negative and the other half is positive, then the positive values are related to the presence of the subject one is interested in, whereas the negative values represent the opposite. Schwartz et al. also suggest that scales that are intended to assess the intensity of a single attribute, for example happiness, should follow a zero-to-positive-value format to emphasize that the question pertains to the absence or presence of this specific attribute, rather than the presence of its opposite. This suggestion is underpinned in an elaborated discussion on happiness as a variable in Kalmijn (2010, Ch. 2). In his thesis, Kalmijn devotes a section to our perspectives on the nature of happiness and satisfaction, the difference between intensity and extensity variables, the polarity of happiness scales and the level of measurement.

The response scale cannot be seen separately from the related leading survey question. Variations in the wording of a question also lead to numerous different survey items. Furthermore, the time frame a question relates to leads to more variations. For example, a question can refer to satisfaction with life over the life time or just at the moment of questioning or for the last 4 weeks. Moreover, a question can contain a keyword such as the word 'happy' in the question "Are you happy with your life?", where the subject can either be explicitly formulated in the response options or not. Likewise a question can be formulated as "Do you feel . . .?" with a keyword only mentioned in the labels of the response options of the related scale.

These are just some examples of the variations in the wording of the questions used in happiness research. Of course there are many more variations one can think of. Each variation will influence the response patterns to a question and can induce structural breaks in the data that can change results dramatically (Cummins and Gullone 2000; Bjørnskov 2010, p. 43; Pudney 2010, p. 6). According to Bjørnskov,

Table 1.1 Classification of survey questions on happiness in the world database of happiness

Aspect	Example	Code
Keyword used	Satisfaction with life	O-SL
Time reference	Currently	c
Method of assessment	Single question	sq
Kind of rating scale	Verbal	v
Length of rating scale	4-step	4
Variant of rating scale	Agree – disagree	a, b,... etc.

a fundamental discussion on this problem, including the framing of life satisfaction questions, has been going on since the 1940s. A comprehensive description of the variations in items and a discussion on these variations is given in, among others, Saris and Gallhofer (2007) and Mazaheri and Theuns (2009). Additionally, a systematic overview of all the variations in survey items on happiness can be found in the collection 'Measures of Happiness' of the WDH. The measures in the WDH are classified by six aspects, see Table 1.1, and the survey questions presented in this book are coded according to this classification.

The Incomparability of Time Series from Different Surveys and Different Time Periods

The Social Indicator Revolution ushered in an era of periodic measurements of several social indicators, among which that for life satisfaction. We will illustrate the diversity in survey items and the comparability problem by using time series on life satisfaction collected in the United States, Japan and The Netherlands. References to these time series and the items used for measuring life satisfaction can be found in the WDH (Veenhoven 2016b).

United States The Gallup organization started measuring life satisfaction in the United States in its Gallup Poll[3] periodically in 1973, asking "In general, are you satisfied or dissatisfied with the way things are going in your own personal life?" using a 2-point verbal scale with the response options labeled 'Satisfied' and 'Dissatisfied'. These same response options were used in the item with the slightly different question "In general, are you satisfied with the way things are going in your personal life at this time?" which Gallup introduced in 2001. At the same time Gallup introduced a second variation on the 1973-item, consisting of the question "In general, how satisfied or dissatisfied are you with the way things are going in your personal life at this time?" and a 4-point verbal scale with the response options labeled 'Very satisfied', 'Somewhat satisfied', 'Somewhat dissatisfied' and 'Very dissatisfied'. These response options were also used in the third variation coming

[3]http://www.gallup.com/products/170987/gallup-analytics.aspx. Assessed 3 February 2016.

with the question "Overall, how satisfied are you with your life…?" which was included in the Gallup Poll in 2005.

Japan In Japan the periodic measurement of life satisfaction started even earlier than in the USA, using a 4-point verbal scale item which was included in the Life-in-Nation survey in 1958. This item consisted of the question "By the way, how do you feel about your life?" and response options labeled 'My life could be better, but on the whole I am satisfied with my current life', 'I am not satisfied with my current life, but it is not too bad to keep more or less on the current level', 'My current life is far from satisfactory', 'I cannot stand my current life'. This item was replaced by a new item in 1964, consisting of the question "How do you feel about your life?" and the response options 'Sufficiently satisfied', 'Rather satisfied, but not sufficiently', 'Fairly dissatisfied' and 'Extremely dissatisfied'. In its turn, this item was replaced in 1970 by the item consisting of the question "How do you feel with life these days" and the response options 'Very satisfied', 'Somewhat satisfied', 'Somewhat dissatisfied' and 'Very dissatisfied'. A replacement of the life satisfaction item in the Life-in-Nation survey followed in 1992, the current item consists of the question "Overall, to what degree are you satisfied with your life these days?" with the response options 'Satisfied', 'Fairly satisfied', 'Somewhat dissatisfied', 'Dissatisfied'.

The Netherlands One of the eldest time series on life satisfaction in The Netherlands comes from a series of measurements by Statistics Netherlands (CBS), which started in 1974 with the launch of the first Life Situation Survey which CBS developed at the request of, and in close collaboration with, The Netherlands Institute for Social Research (SCP). The item used for these measurements was the 5-point verbal scale item consisting of the question "To what extent are you satisfied with the life you currently" with the response options 'Extraordinarily satisfied', 'Very satisfied', 'Satisfied', 'Fairly satisfied' and 'Not very satisfied'. This item was used in changing surveys by both SCP and CBS with different periodicities over a period of almost 40 years (DeJonge 2009): CBS used the item for life satisfaction until 2010. After having conducted a split-half experiment in 2012, in which a verbal and a numerical scale were used to measure life satisfaction, CBS decided to change to a 10-point numerical response scale (Van Beuningen et al. 2014). The SCP used the verbal scale until 2002 when it changed to a 10-point numerical scale for life satisfaction.

The Rank Method In survey research it is common practice to assign ranks to the response options of a discrete scale to calculate a sample mean, regardless of the semantics of the wording used to label the options. The sample mean is accordingly calculated as the weighted average of the ranks of the response options using the relative frequencies as weights. In this common practice, denoted the Rank Method, it is implicitly assumed that equivalent response options in equivalent scales are evaluated identically and that the response options are equally distanced regardless of the topic of concern. The value range assigned to the words by which a response option is labeled, however, heavily depends on the context of the scale as does the

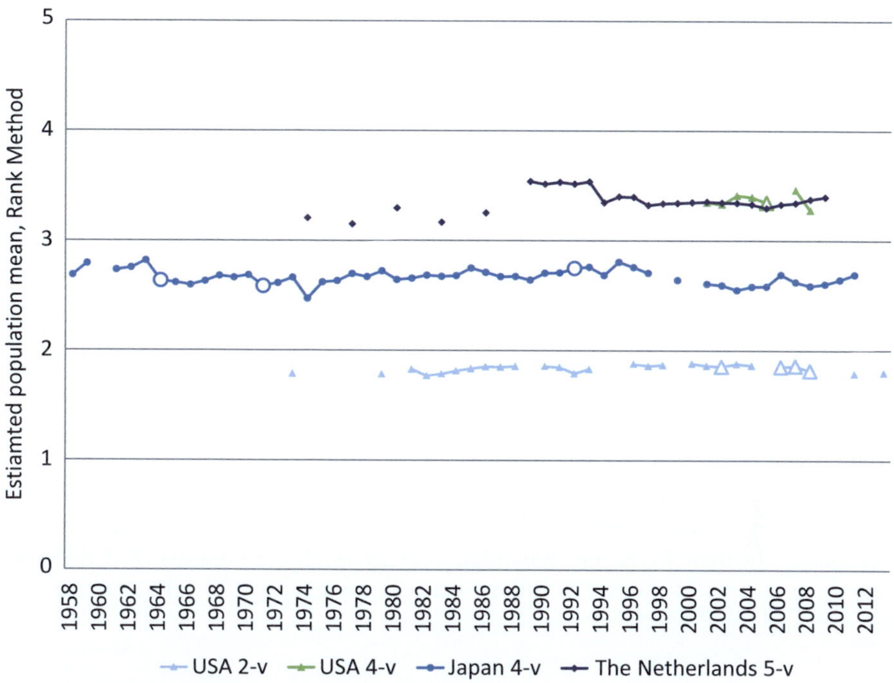

Fig. 1.1 Mean life satisfaction in the USA, Japan and The Netherlands based on the Rank Method

distance between two consecutive response options, see Chap. 5. This notion emphasizes the difficulty of comparing the outcomes of different surveys.

There are a number of other problems for trend analysis than just the ones mentioned above that complicate the comparability of survey outcomes and it is difficult to pool these results into long, consistent time series. Much of this becomes clear if we look at Fig. 1.1, in which time series of a sample mean according to the Rank Method, are presented for the previously described time series on life satisfaction in the United States, Japan and The Netherlands. In the legend of Fig. 1.1 the number of response options used is given, followed by '-v' for verbal. Any change in the survey item used is marked in the time series by a large marker with no colour inside.

As can be seen from Fig. 1.1 it is obvious that there are considerable scale-effects if the Rank Method is applied to calculate a sample mean. The means according to the Rank Method for the three countries differ considerably, due to the differences in the number of response options,. An exception to this are the means based on the 4-point scales used in the USA and the means based on the 5-point scale used in The Netherlands which come very close. This is, however, counterintuitive given the difference in the number of the response options used, it is likely that it can be attributed to the labeling of the response options used. This labeling causes respondents who are satisfied with their life to select a response option with an, on average, relative high rank when they have to rate their life satisfaction on the 4-point scale used in the USA and to select a response option with an, on average, relatively low rank when they have to rate their life satisfaction on the 5-point scale used in The Netherlands, see Chap. 5. The same four response options as those used in the USA, were employed in Japan from 1970 to 1991 in combination with a similar question. This resulted in much lower means for Japan than for the USA. This could mean that life satisfaction in Japan is on average lower than in the USA, but also, that the Japanese assign a different value range to the same response options.

Another fact which has to be taken into account when improving the comparability of time series is the periodicity of measurement which will differ per survey and which has changed over the course of time for some surveys. This may cause discontinuities, but also changes in the mode of surveying result in discontinuities in the time series, see the data for the time series in The Netherlands in Fig. 1.1. We will go into more detail on this in Chap. 11.

The above are just some of the issues that have to be addressed when searching for causes of incomparability when dealing with mixed survey data, but they certainly contribute to our understanding that the pooling of outcomes of different survey items into long consistent time series is not a straightforward exercise.

Conventional Scale Transformation Methods for Items from Different Surveys

The limited uniformity of survey items and the other problems that affect the comparability of survey results reduces our ability to accumulate knowledge of such items and limits our analyses of trends. To deal with this problem calls for methods to transform ratings on different scales to attain comparable results and to correct for effects of changes in measurements and other influencing factors. Several methods have been developed to transform ratings on different response scales to a common one, typically a scale ranging from 0 to 10. Some of these scale transformation methods are applied in the World Database of Happiness, in particular in its collection of 'Happiness in Nations' (Veenhoven 2016b). In this section we describe some of the conventional methods used and explain why they fall short as a means to overcome the comparability problem caused by the non-uniformity of survey items.

Linear Stretch

A simple and commonly used conventional transformation method is the Linear Stretch Method, an early version of which was in use almost a century ago (Hull

1922). The Linear Stretch Method is most applicable for questions that use a numerical response scale. Scales with five or seven response options are typically stretched to obtain a common range for example from 0 to 10. This is done in such a way that the number corresponding to the response option representing the worst case in the scale is always projected onto 0 and the number representing the best case in the scale onto the highest value of the range, and all the intermediate options are given equally distanced numbers in between: for a 5-point verbal scale the transformation to a 0–10 scale according to this method results in {0.0; 2.5; 5.0; 7.5; 10.0}. The sample mean after transformation of the scale follows from the conventional Weighted Average Approach[4] according to which the mean is equal to the sum of the - transformed - values of all response options multiplied by their respective measured relative frequencies. When a verbal scale has to be transformed in this way, an initial step is to assign numerical values to verbal response options, typically using consecutive numbers, such as four for the happiest option on a four-step scale and one for the least happy option.

The Linear Stretch Method has many serious disadvantages. The two most prominent of these disadvantages are one, the assumption made that the distances between the response options are equal, and two, even more problematically, the assumption that the labeling of the response options is irrelevant to the analysis, though not for the respondent. Despite these disadvantages, the Linear Stretch Method is still applied, for example it is used in the World Database of Happiness for numerical scales with at least seven points to transform them to comparable scales with a 0–10 range. The effect of scale transformation using the Linear Stretch Method depending on the number of response options of the primary scale is discussed in depth in Batz et al. (2015).

The Percentage of Scale Maximum Another example of where the Linear Stretch Method is applied is in the Percentage of Scale Maximum (%SM) Method developed by Cummins (1997, 2003). In this method Likert scale data are transformed to a standard form with a range from 0 to 100. In the %SM-method a score of '0' is given to the lowest scale anchor up to 'k' to represent the highest scale anchor. Any mean score on this scale can subsequently be converted into %SM units by converting the score into a percentage of the scale maximum value as: %SM = (mean score/k)*100.

The %SM-method encounters the same disadvantages as mentioned above for the Linear Stretch Method, since it is based on a simple linear relationship between the response options and disregards their labeling. A practical and illustrative example of the discrepancy in outcomes which might occur when the %SM-method is applied to survey results for life satisfaction based on different response scales is given in DeJonge et al. (2015, p. 82).

---

[4]The Weighted Average Approach is a generalization of the Rank Method, but does not require that the numbers assigned to the response options are equal to the ranks of these response options to calculate a sample mean.

Semantic Judgment of Fixed Word Value

Several attempts have been made in the course of happiness research to develop better methods to cope with the heterogeneity in response scales. What many of these alternative methods have in common is that they make use of expert ratings (Veenhoven 1993; Bălţătescu 2002; Lim 2008) where a group of experts rate the verbal labels of response options on a common numerical scale.

An early example of such a method is that of Jones and Thurstone (1955) who requested approximately 900 respondents to rate 51 verbal qualifications on a 9-point Likert scale separately. A value on a common interval scale and a standard deviation were calculated for each qualification. The result was a list of the 51 qualifications ordered on the basis of their value on the common interval scale. Another illustration of this method can be found in the work done by Lodge (1981). We have classified this method as the Semantic Judgment of Fixed Word Value Method, and it is also applied in the World Database of Happiness to obtain comparable average scores. Veenhoven (1993) and 12 co-workers rated the degree of happiness denoted by the verbal labels of 29 commonly used survey items on a numerical 0–10 scale. For example, the label 'Very happy' was an option in eight of the 29 items and was given a rating varying from 9.2 to 9.4 resulting in an overall mean of 9.3, whereas for the label 'Not very happy' an overall mean of 3.7 was found. To this day, these results are used to transform responses in the WDH with scales for which linear stretching falls short.

The Semantic Judgment of Fixed Word Value Method overcomes the disadvantages of presumed equidistance and the neglecting of the labels that are associated with the Linear Stretch Method. The Semantic Judgment of Fixed Word Value Method, however, also has some weak points. Kalmijn (2010, p. 118) mentions that the fixed values applied in the World Database of Happiness:

- are based on expert judgments that do not necessarily reflect the views of non-expert respondents
- have been rated by Dutch experts on basis of the English version of the questions, thus implicitly assuming that the feelings associated with an item are not affected by its translation from Dutch into English
- do not take into account the phrasing of the lead question, nor the number and the labels of the alternative response options and their position on the scale

Some Words on Methods to Correct for Response Heterogeneity at the Individual Level

In this book we focus on the comparability of existing survey data that have been collected over the years using different survey items on the same topic in different surveys. These survey items, and the surveys they come from, may still be in use, but this is not necessarily the case. Often, the only information that is available for a given survey item, is the survey it was employed in, the mode of surveying, the period of data collection, the number of respondents, the sample size and the population this sample was drawn from, the language used, the country and, last but not least, the frequency distribution of the response. As far as information at the level of an individual respondent is available, this may differ from survey to survey and is therefore often not comparable between surveys. The available data is sufficient for the application of the conventional transformation methods described in section "Conventional scale transformation methods for items from different surveys". The comparability intended using these methods is at the aggregate level of the mean and standard deviation within a population or subgroups of the population, thus at the macro and meso level. With this book we intent to provide tools and insights into how to make better use of existing survey data which has been collected across countries and in different languages over time and which may have been completed with newly collected data.

The problem of comparability between countries and subgroups of the population caused by the differential use of response scales by survey respondents is also studied in an adjacent, flourishing discipline of ongoing research in the field of for example health science or economics about which a large body of literature is available. In this research discipline methods have and are being developed and applied to adjust survey results for this heterogeneity in reporting behaviour, on basis of the characteristics of the individual respondents. These methods are applicable for adjusting the survey results for one or more survey items which are included in the same survey by which the characteristics of individual respondents are collected, which may be employed in different languages and countries. Much of this literature about the methods used to make data comparable and their application can be found within the field of health sciences. We mention some of these methods for the interested reader, but do not go into details, as this kind of adjustment of survey data at the individual level fall outside the scope of this book. A simple method introduced in the mid nineteenhundreds is Ridit-analysis[5] (Bross 1958; Donaldson 1998; Uwawunkonye and Anaene 2013). In this method the frequency distribution for a, to be specified, group of respondents is used to derive reference scores which are used to compare with the results for other groups of respondents. A more advanced method is that where ratings on a Visual Analogue Scale (VAS)[6] are compared to multi-item measures (McDowell 2006). An advanced example of this has been developed by the EuroQol Group[7]: the widely used EQ-5D self-report questionnaire which measures quality of life on five

[5]Ridit stands for *Relative to an Identified Distribution Integral Transformation.*

[6]A VAS is a measurement instrument used to ask respondents to specify their level of agreement with a statement on a subjective topic by indicating a position along a continuous line between two end-points.

[7]A network of international multidisciplinary researchers committed to the measurement of health-related quality of life, www.euroqol.org.

dimensions and a VAS (Szende et al. 2007, 2014). A third and recently method is the Vignettes Method (Kapteyn et al. 2007; Valentine et al. 2015). In this method respondents have to, for example, rate their own life satisfaction and, on the same scale, that of several hypothetical people presented to the respondents using vignette descriptions of the conditions faced by these characters. The vignette evaluations are then used to identify the differences between the response scales. Using scales in one country as a benchmark, the distribution of evaluations in other countries can then be adjusted by evaluating the responses using the benchmark scale.

To our knowledge, these methods to correct for response heterogeneity at the individual level are not suitable for retroactive application.

The Need for Further Innovation

The weaknesses of the early transformation methods to reduce the response heterogeneity described in section "Conventional scale transformation methods for items from different surveys" also appear when the transformed scores are compared to average ratings on 0–10 numerical scales in the same country in the same year (Kalmijn et al. 2011). All the weaknesses of these conventional methods have driven further innovations in the field of making data comparable and it is this which will be discussed in this book.

References

Andrews, F. M., & Withey, S. B. (1976). *Social indicator of well-being, Americans' perceptions of life quality*. New York: Plenum Press.

Bălţătescu, S. (2002). *Problems of transforming scales of life satisfaction*. Euromodule workshop, Berlin. Retrieved January 29, 2014, http://worlddatabaseofhappiness.eur.nl-hap_bib-freetexts-baltatescu_sm_2002A.pdf

Batz, C., Parrigon, S. & Tay, L. (2015). The impact of scale transformations on National subjective well-being scores. Social Indicators Research, Published online: 04 Sep 2015. doi: 10.1007/s11205-015-1088-1

Bjørnskov, C. (2010). How comparable are the gallup world poll life satisfaction data? *Journal of Happiness Studies, 11*, 41–60. doi:10.1007/s10902-008-9121-6.

Bross, I. D. J. (1958). How to use ridit analysis. *Biometrics, 14*, 18–38.

Campbell, A., Converse, P. E., & Rodgers, W. L. (1976). *The quality of American life. Perceptions, evaluations, and satisfactions*. New York: Russel Sage Foundation. Available at: http://babel.hathitrust.org/cgi/pt?id=mdp.39015071884634;view=2up;seq=6.

Cummins, R. A. (1997). *The comprehensive quality of life scale – intellectual-cognitive disability (ComQol-I5)* (5th ed.). Melbourne: School of Psychology, Deakin University.

Cummins, R. A. & Gullone, E. (2000). *Why we should not use 5-point Likert scales: The case for subjective quality of life measurement*. Proceedings, second international conference on quality of life in cities (pp. 74–93). Singapore: National University of Singapore

Cummins, R. A. (2003). Normative life satisfaction: Measurement issues and homeostatic model. *Social Indicators Research, 64*, 225–240.

DeJonge, T. (2009). *The state of play in measuring SWB in the Netherlands*. Paper for the OECD meeting Measuring subjective well-being: An opportunity for National Statistical Offices?, Florence, Italy. Retrieved January 29, 2016, Available at: http://worlddatabaseofhappiness.eur.nl/hap_bib/freetexts/dejonge_t_2009a.pdf

DeJonge, T., Veenhoven, R., & Arends, L. R. (2015). 'Very Happy' is not always equally happy on the meaning of verbal response options in survey questions. *Journal of Happiness Studies, 16*(1), 77–101. doi:10.1007-s10902-013-9497-9.

Diener, E., & Diener, C. (1996). Most people are happy. *Psychological Science, 7*, 181–185.

Donaldson, G. W. (1998). Ridit scores for analysis and interpretation of ordinal pain data. *European Journal of Pain, 2*, 221–227.

Frijters, P., Johnston, D. W., & Shields, M. A. (2008). *Happiness dynamics with quarterly life event data* (IZA Discussion Paper No. 3604).

Gallup (2016). *Understanding how gallup uses the Cantril scale*. Retrieved January 29, 2016, http://www.gallup.com/poll/122453/understanding-gallup-uses-cantril-scale.aspx

Guven, C., Senik, C., & Stichnoth, H. (2011). *You can't be happier than your wife. Happiness gaps and divorce* (Paris School of Economics, Working Paper No. 2011–01, halshs-00555427).

Hull, C. L. (1922). The conversion of test scores into series which shall have any assigned mean and degree of dispersion. *Journal of Applied Psychology, 6*(3), 298–300.

Jones, L. V., & Thurstone, L. L. (1955). The psychophysics of semantics. An experimental investigation. *The Journal of Applied Psychology, 39*(1), 31–36.

Kalmijn, W. M. (2010). *Quantification of happiness inequality*. Dissertation, Erasmus University Rotterdam, The Netherlands. Enschede: Ipskamp Drukkers. Available at http://repub.eur.nl/pub/21777

Kalmijn, W. M., Arends, L. R., & Veenhoven, R. (2011). Happiness scale interval study, methodological considerations. *Social Indicators Research, 102*(3), 497–515. doi:10.1007/s11205-010-9688-2.

Kapteyn, A., Smith, J. P., & van Soest, A. (2007). Vignettes and self-reports of work disability in the United States and the Netherlands. *American Economic Review, 97*(1), 461–473.

Lee, H., Kim, K. D., & Shin, D. C. (1982). Perceptions of quality of life in an industrializing country: The case of the Republic of Korea. *Social Indicators Research, 10*, 297–317. doi:10.1007/BF00301097.

Lim, H. E. (2008). The use of different happiness rating scales: Bias and comparison problem? *Social Indicators Research, 87*, 259–267. doi:10.1007/s11205-007-9171-x.

Lodge, M. (1981). Magnitude scaling: Quantitative measurement of opinions. Beverly Hills: Sage Publications, Series Quantitative applications in the social sciences, ISSN 0149-192X; 07-025. doi: 10.4135/9781412984874

Mazaheri, M., & Theuns, P. (2009). Effects of varying response formats on self-ratings of life-satisfaction. *Social Indicators Research, 90*, 381–395. doi:10.1007/s11205-008-9263-2.

McDowell, I. (2006). *Measuring health. A guide to rating scales and questionnaires* (3rd ed.). Oxford: Oxford University Press. http://a4ebm.org/sites/default/files/Measuring%20Health.pdf.

Pudney, S. (2010). *An experimental analysis of the impact of survey design on measures and models of subjective wellbeing* (ISER Working Paper Series, 2010–20). Economic & Social Research Council. Retrieved February 3, 2016, www.iser.essex.ac.uk/research/publications/working-papers/iser/2010-20.pdf

Sangster, R. L., Willits, F. K., Saltiel, J., Lorenz, F. O., & Rockwood, T. H. (2001). *The effect of numerical labels on response scales*. Article presented at the Annual Meeting of the American Statistical Association, Atlanta. http://www.bls.gov-osmr-pdf-st010120.pdf

Saris, W. E. & Gallhofer, I. N. (2007). *Design, evaluation, and analysis of questionnaires for survey research*(Wiley series in survey methodology). New York: Wiley-Interscience. ISBN 978-0-470-11495-7, e-ISBN 978-0-470-16519-5

Schwarz, N., Knauper, B., Hippler, H. J., Noelle-Neumann, E., & Clark, W. (1991). Rating scales: Numeric values may change the meaning of scale labels. *The Public Opinion Quarterly*, 55, 570–582. http://www.jstor.org-stable-2749407

Szende, A., Oppe, M., & Devlin, N. (Eds.). (2007). *EQ-5D value sets. Inventory, comparative review and user guide*. Dordrecht: Springer.

Szende, A., Janssen, B., & Cabases, J. (Eds.). (2014). *Self-reported population health: An international perspective based on EQ-5D*. Dordrecht: Springer. doi:10.1007/978-94-007-7596-1.

Uwawunkonye, E. G., & Anaene, O. I. C. (2013). A comparative study between ridit and modified ridit analysis. *American Journal of Theoretical and Applied Statistics, 2*(6), 248–254. doi:10.11648/j.ajtas.20130206.23.

Valentine, N., Verdes-Tennant, & Bonsel, G. (2015). Health systems' responsiveness and reporting behaviour: Multilevel analysis of the influence of individual-level factors in 64 countries. *Social Science & Medicine, 138*, 152–160.

van Beuningen, J., van der Houwen, K., & Moonen, L. (2014). *Measuring well-being, an analysis of different response scales* (Discussion Paper, Statistics Netherlands). Retrieved July 20, 2015, http://www.cbs.nl-NR-rdonlyres-FF644A99-580C-4D7E-B214-BEE54A947D46-0-Measuringwellbeing.pdf

Veenhoven, R. (1984). *Databook of happiness*. Dordrecht: Reidel Publishing. ISBN 90-277-1793-1

Veenhoven, R. (1993). Happiness in nations, subjective appreciation of life in 56 nations, 1946–1992. *Studies in Social-Cultural Transformation*, 2. Risbo, Erasmus University Rotterdam, Netherlands. Available at: https://personal.eur.nl/veenhoven/Pub1990s/93b-con.html

Veenhoven, R. (2011). *World database of happiness, example of a focused 'Findings Archive'* (RatSWD, Working Paper Series, Working Paper, 169). Retrieved January 29, 2016, http://www.ratswd.de/download/RatSWD_WP_2011/RatSWD_WP_169.pdf

Veenhoven, R. (2016a). *Measures of happiness*. World Database of happiness, Erasmus University Rotterdam. Available at: http://worlddatabaseofhappiness.eur.nl/hap_quer/hqi_fp.htm

Veenhoven, R. (2016b). *Happiness in Nations*. World Database of Happiness, Erasmus University Rotterdam. Available at: http://worlddatabaseofhappiness.eur.nl/hap_nat/nat_fp.php?mode=1

Part II
Innovation 1: The Happiness Scale Interval Study

Chapter 2
The Happiness Scale Interval Study

Introduction to the Happiness Scale Interval Study

Veenhoven (2008) started the Happiness Scale Interval Study (HSIS) to counter the shortcomings of the Semantic Judgment of Fixed Word Value Method. This study was set up to look at survey questions on happiness using verbal response options, such as 'Very happy' and 'Pretty happy' to determine consistently what degrees of happiness are denoted by such terms when used in particular questions and different languages. The main aim of the HSIS is to improve the comparison of happiness across nations. Therefore, the items included in the HSIS are restricted to those that have been applied in studies of general populations in nations. Since it came into existence the HSIS has been conducted in a number of countries. A complete list of all items ever considered since the start of the study in 2005 can be found on the website of the World Database of Happiness, in the section 'Scale Interval Study'. In the HSIS persons who are referred to as 'judges' are asked to rate the degree of happiness denoted by each of the verbal response options in the context of the full item. The judges are asked to identify the interval on a 0–10 range that corresponds to a verbal response option such as 'Very happy' using a web-based Scale Interval Recorder (Veenhoven and Hermus 2006). This method is discussed in detail in (Kalmijn 2010; Kalmijn et al. 2011) and we will refer to it as the Scale Interval Method.

The Scale Interval Recorder

A series of survey items is presented on a computer screen to judges. Items are presented sequentially on the left side of the screen and each item presented consists of a question and its corresponding verbal response scale with options given in the judges' mother tongue. A screen shot of the Scale Interval Recorder from the trial

T. de Jonge et al., *Diversity in Survey Questions on the Same Topic*, Social Indicators Research Series 68, DOI 10.1007/978-3-319-53261-5_2

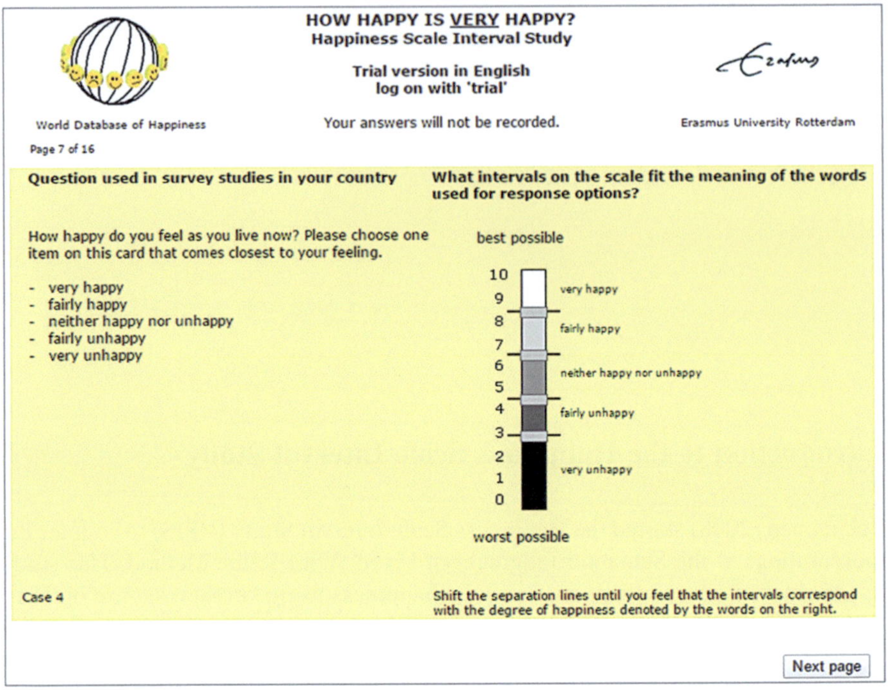

Fig. 2.1 Screenshot of the scale interval recorder

version[1] in English which is available in the WDH is given in Fig. 2.1. On the right side of the screen a vertical bar scale is displayed with small horizontal sliders on it, the number of which is equal to the number of response options of the scale minus one. The judges have to shift the sliders until they feel that the intervals on the vertical bar correspond to the meaning of the words as used for the verbal response options. Note, the response options that are displayed next to the bar move simultaneously with the sliders to the level of the mid-interval value of each interval. Looking at Fig. 2.1 it can be seen that the extremes of the numerical bar scale are labeled 'Worst possible' and 'Best possible'. In the terminology of Saris and Gallhofer (2007) these labels are called 'fixed reference points'. What worst and what best means, is left to the interpretation of the judges. The labeling of the extremes is thus semi-abstract which makes them applicable to all questions presented to the judges and independent of the subject of an individual question. An additional advantage of this semi-abstract labeling is that a judgment is not influenced by the wording used for the labels of both extremes of the continuum.

[1] http://www.risbo.org/fsw/english-trial/

Difference with Conventional Methods for Scale Transformation

The approach to scale transformation used in the HSIS differs essentially from that used in the Linear Stretch Method and the Semantic Judgment of Fixed Word Value Method, as the response options in the primary scale are not considered to be discrete points, but to be intervals each representing a part of the continuum from 0 to 10 where the perception of happiness can be found. This complies with the assumption that attitudes fall along a single, latent continuum which is commonly discretized for the convenience of surveying methods (Scherpenzeel 1999, p. 16; Saris and Gallhofer 2007, p. 19; Studer 2011, p. 1). In the Happiness Scale Interval Study each response option is judged in the context of the other response options of the scale and this approach is illustrative of the Scale Interval Method.

Three Scale Transformation Methods Applied to Empirical Data

To illustrate how the three methods, Linear Stretch, Semantic Judgment of Fixed Word Value and Scale Interval, are used we selected two survey items used to measure life satisfaction in The Netherlands. The first of these items is the item from Statistics Netherlands (CBS) that we introduced in Chap. 1. The second item comes from the Eurobarometer (EB), a series of public opinion surveys conducted in the member states of the European Union regularly on behalf of the European Commission which dates back to 1973. The standard version of the EB has, almost without exception, a spring wave and an autumn wave for every year since then (Schmitt et al. 2008; European Commission 2012a, b, 2013–2015). The items are summarized in Table 2.1, which also includes their WDH classification code according to Table 1.1.

The CBS item has an asymmetric response scale with five options. The EB item has a symmetric response scale without a neutral midpoint and four options. The two items together comprise six response options, three of which are included in both items. The transformation of the response scales of the items to a scale from 0 to 10 according to each of the three transformation methods is depicted in Fig. 2.2.

From Fig. 2.2 it can be seen that in the Linear Stretch Method the anchor points of both primary scales are pinned to 0 and 10 and that all the other response options are equally spaced in between. When the Linear Stretch Method is applied the response option ‘Fairly satisfied’ of the 5-point scale is assigned the transformed value 2.5, whereas this option for the 4-point scale gets a transformed value of 6.7. This large difference between the values 2.5 and 6.7 is elucidatory for the fact that the wordings of the response options are neglected when the Linear Stretch Method is applied.

Table 2.1 Survey items on satisfaction with life used in The Netherlands in two surveys

Item code survey	Question	Response options	Frequencies 2008
O-SLL-c-sq-v-5-d CBS	To what extent are you satisfied with the life you currently lead?	Extraordinarily satisfied	8.4%
		Very satisfied	35.5%
		Satisfied	45.1%
		Fairly satisfied	7.6%
		Not very satisfied	3.4%
O-SLL-u-sq-v-4-b EB	On the whole how satisfied are you with the life you lead?	Very satisfied	51.5%
		Fairly satisfied	44.8%
		Not very satisfied	3.1%
		Not at all satisfied	0.6%

If the Semantic Judgment of Fixed Word Value Method is applied the results are entirely different. The value of a label such as ‘Fairly satisfied’ is fixed in this method and equal to 6.5 according to the Dutch experts, however, from Fig. 2.2 it can also be seen that the Semantic Judgment of Fixed Word Value Method treats each response option as isolated from the number and the wording of the other options and thus does not take into account the context of the scale.

As can be seen in the Scale Interval Method the assumption of equal distances between response options and the idea that a fixed value applies to a label of a response option irrespective of the labeling of the other options is abandoned. If we consider the response option ‘Fairly satisfied’ once more, we can see that this option is assigned the interval 3.6–5.3 for the 5-point scale, with a mid-interval value equal to 4.5 and a length of 1.7. For the 4-point scale the interval for this option ranges from 5.3 to 7.9, with a mid-interval value of 6.6 and a length of 2.6.

The Three Transformation Methods and the Comparability Problem

At the start of the Happiness Scale Interval Study in the Scale Interval Method a sample mean after transformation of the primary scale was based on the conventional Weighted Average Approach according to which the mean is equal to the sum of the mid-interval values of all intervals of the transformed scale, each of which values is weighted with its corresponding relative frequency. This is analogous to how this is done in the Linear Stretch Method and the Semantic Judgment of Fixed Word Value Method. A comparison of the results obtained using these three scale transformation methods is given in Table 2.2.

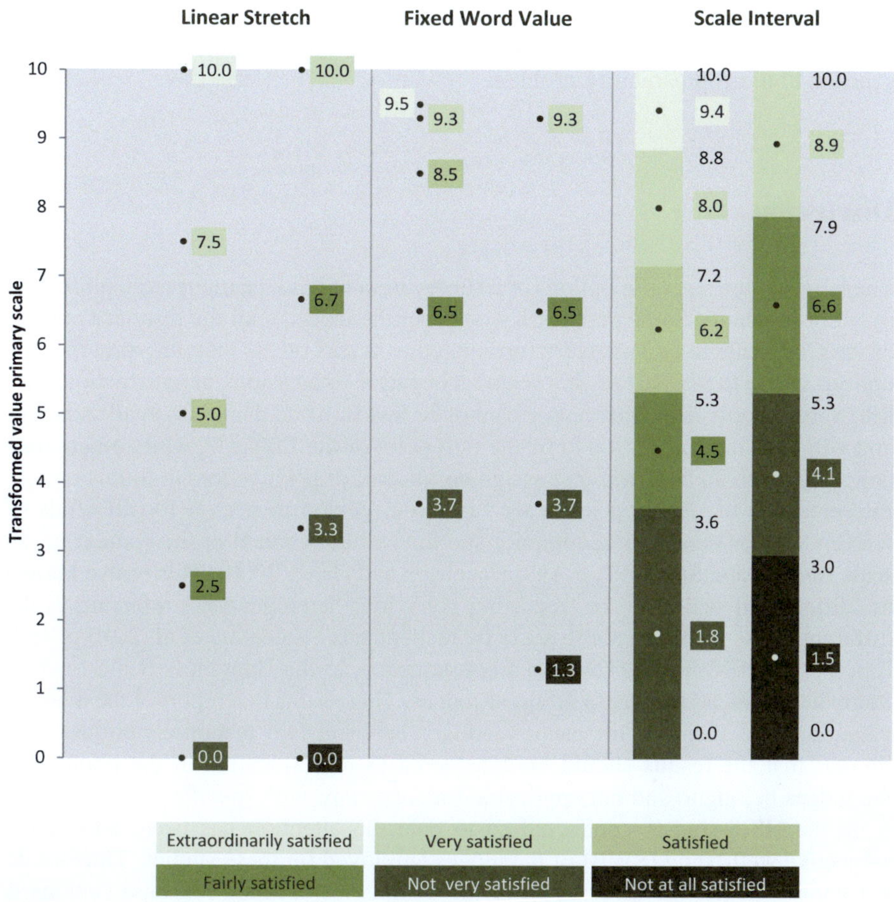

Fig. 2.2 Comparison of transformations using three methods

Table 2.2 Transformed means obtained using different transformation methods (frequencies 2008)

Item code survey	Linear stretch	Semantic judgment of fixed word value	Scale interval
O-SLL-c-sq-v-5-d CBS	5.9	8.6	6.9
O-SLL-u-sq-v-4-b EB	8.2	7.8	7.7

The survey items from CBS and the EB address more or less the same topic and mainly differ in the response scales. The results for each item are assumed to be representative for the Dutch population and therefore one would expect that, given that a transformation method is applied, the transformed means for 2008 would be equal. This is clearly not the case. The difference of 2.3 between the transformed means of 5.9 and 8.2 based on the Linear Stretch Method is most striking. Taking these results it is obvious that none of the three transformation methods offers a solution to the comparability problem.

Discussion

The labels of the response options of a survey item will not be interpreted uniformly by all respondents. Some people may consider the labels of all the response options of the CBS scale to be positively formulated, whereas others may interpret the two options at the lower part of this scale as negative expressions of satisfaction with life. Some people may believe one cannot be less satisfied than 'Not at all satisfied' and will consider this option to be the null point of the EB scale, while others may believe things can be worse and assign an interval of positive length to this option. Interpretation of semantic intervals vary from person to person for all kinds of reasons such as personality, ethnicity and the cultural context or the context of the scale (Diener and Suh 1997, p. 197; Hazelrigg and Hardy 2000). This is also known as 'differential scale use' or 'reporting behaviour heterogeneity', referring to the differential use of the response scale by respondents (Valentine et al. 2015 p. 153; Exton et al. 2015, pp. 20–24). As a consequence, in the Happiness Scale Interval Study items are assessed by a group of judges. This results in a report of the average value and the variance for each boundary between two response options. This implies that the results should be considered as representative of the population the judges belong to and not applicable for subgroups with specific characteristics.

In the HSIS-studies conducted so to date, no attention has been paid to the subjective well-being (SWB) of the judges employed for these studies. Thus we do not know whether the assessment of the boundaries between response options is affected by the judges' SWB. It is desirable to set up an HSIS-study to investigate this, as has been recommended by Kalmijn (2010, p. 179) previously.

All of the three transformation methods have in common that a discrete primary scale is transformed into a discrete secondary scale and that the sample mean is calculated on the basis of all ratings of this 'secondary scale'. This sample mean is then adopted as the estimator of the mean happiness value of the happiness distribution in the population. The variance and standard deviation of the latter distribution are estimated accordingly. The three methods also have in common that they do not offer a solution to the comparability problem as we have shown in Table 2.2.

Solving the comparability problem requires another approach, which we will tackle in more detail in Chap. 7 onwards. The Scale Interval Method, however, does offer some interesting applications which allow us a perspective on the size of the comparability problem. These applications will be discussed in Chaps. 4, 5, and 6.

References

Diener, E., & Suh, E. (1997). Measuring quality of life: Economic, social and subjective indicators. *Social Indicators Research, 40*, 189–216.

European Commission. (2012a). Brussels. European Opinion Research Group (EORG). GESIS Data Archive, Cologne. *Eurobarometer 57.1 (Mar–May 2002),* ZA3639 Data file Version 1.0.1. doi:10.4232/1.10949; *Eurobarometer 58.1 (Oct–Nov 2002),* ZA3693 Data file Version 1.0.1. doi:10.4232/1.10953; *Eurobarometer 60.1 (Oct–Nov 2003)*, ZA3938 Data file Version 1.0.1. doi:10.4232/1.10958; *Eurobarometer 62.0 (Oct–Nov 2004)*, ZA4229 Data file Version 1.1.0. doi:10.4232/1.10962.

European Commission. (2012b). Brussels. TNS opinion & social [producer]. GESIS Data Archive, Cologne. *Eurobarometer 63.4 (May–Jun 2005)*, ZA4411 Data file Version 1.1.0. doi:10.4232/1.10968; *Eurobarometer 64.2 (Oct–Nov 2005)*, ZA4414 Data file Version 1.1.0. doi:10.4232/1.10970; *Eurobarometer 65.2 (Mar–May 2006)*, ZA4506 Data file Version 1.0.1. doi:10.4232/1.10974; *Eurobarometer 66.1 (Sep–Oct 2006)*, ZA4526 Data file Version 1.0.1. doi:10.4232/1.10980; *Eurobarometer 66.3 (Nov–Dec 2006)*, ZA4528 Data file Version 2.0.1. doi:10.4232/1.10982; *Eurobarometer 67.2 (Apr–May 2007)*, ZA4530 Data file Version 2.1.0. doi:10.4232/1.10984; *Eurobarometer 68.1 (Sep–Nov 2007)*, ZA4565 Data file Version 4.0.1. doi:10.4232/1.10988; *Eurobarometer 70.1 (Oct–Nov 2008)*, ZA4819 Data file Version 3.0.2. doi:10.4232/1.10989; *Eurobarometer 71.2 (May–Jun 2009)*, ZA4972 Data file Version 3.0.2. doi:10.4232/1.10990; *Eurobarometer 72.4 (Oct–Nov 2009)*, ZA4994 Data file Version 3.0.0. doi:10.4232/1.11141; *Eurobarometer 73.4 (May 2010)*, ZA5234 Data file Version 2.0.1. doi:10.4232/1.11479; *Eurobarometer 76.3 (2011)*, ZA5567 Data file Version 1.0.0. doi:10.4232/1.11448.

European Commission. (2013–2015). Brussels. TNS opinion & social [producer]. GESIS Data Archive, Cologne. *Eurobarometer 69.2 (Mar–May 2008)*, ZA4744 Data file Version 5.0.0. doi:10.4232/1.11755; *Eurobarometer 71.1 (Jan–Feb 2009)*, ZA4971 Data file Version 4.0.0. doi:10.4232/1.11756; *Eurobarometer 74.2 (2010)*, ZA5449 Data file Version 2.2.0. doi:10.4232/1.11626; *Eurobarometer 75.3 (2011)*, ZA5481 Data file Version 2.0.0. doi:10.4232/1.11768; *Eurobarometer 75.4 (2011)*, ZA5564 Data file Version 3.0.0. doi:10.4232/1.11769; *Eurobarometer 77.3 (2012)*, ZA5612 Data file Version 1.0.0. doi:10.4232/1.11558; *Eurobarometer 77.4 (2012)*, ZA5613 Data file Version 2.0.0. doi:10.4232/1.11697; *Eurobarometer 78.1 (2012)*, ZA5685 Data file Version 1.0.0. doi:10.4232/1.11706 *Eurobarometer 79.3 (2013)*, ZA5689 Data file Version 1.1.0. doi:10.4232/1.12445; *Eurobarometer 80.1 (2013)*, ZA5876 Data file Version 1.0.0. doi:10.4232/1.11881; *Eurobarometer 81.2 (2014)*, ZA5913 Data file Version 1.0.0. doi:10.4232/1.12172; *Eurobarometer 81.4 (2014)*, ZA5928 Data file Version 2.0.0. doi:10.4232/1.12201; *Eurobarometer 82.3 (2014)*, ZA5932 Data file Version 2.0.1. doi:10.4232/1.12259; *Eurobarometer 83.1 (2015)*, ZA5964 Data file Version 1.0.0. doi:10.4232/1.12340; *Eurobarometer 83.3 (2015)*, ZA5998 Data file Version 1.0.0. doi:10.4232/1.12356.

Exton, C., Smith, C., & Vandendriessche, D. (2015). *Comparing happiness across countries: Does culture matter?* (OECD Statistics Working Papers, 2015/04). OECD Publishing, Paris. doi:10.1787/18152031. Retrieved February 15, 2016, http://www.oecd-ilibrary.org/economics/comparing-happiness-across-the-world_5jrqppzd9bs2-en?crawler=true

Hazelrigg, L. E., & Hardy, M. A. (2000). Scaling the semantics of satisfaction. *Social Indicators Research, 49*(2), 147–180. doi:10.1023/A:1006937713249.

Kalmijn, W.M. (2010). *Quantification of happiness inequality*. Dissertation, Erasmus University Rotterdam, The Netherlands. Enschede: Ipskamp Drukkers. Available at http://repub.eur.nl/pub/21777

Kalmijn, W. M., Arends, L. R., & Veenhoven, R. (2011). Happiness scale interval study, methodological considerations. *Social Indicators Research, 102*(3), 497–515. doi:10.1007/s11205-010-9688-2.

Saris, W. E., & Gallhofer, I. N. (2007). *Design, evaluation, and analysis of questionnaires for survey research* (Wiley series in survey methodology). New York: Wiley-Interscience. ISBN 978-0-470-11495-7, e-ISBN 978-0-470-16519-5.

Scherpenzeel, A. (1999). *Why use 11-point scales? Documentation of the Swiss Household Panel.* http://forscenter.ch-en-our-surveys-swiss-household-panel-documentationfaq-methods-varia-. Accessed May 2014.

Schmitt, H., Scholz, E., Leim, I., & Moschner, M. (2008). *The Mannheim eurobarometer trend file 1970–2002* (ed. 2.00). European Commission [Principal investigator]. GESIS Data Archive, Cologne. ZA3521 Data file Version 2.0.1. doi: 10.4232/1.10074.

Studer, R. (2011). *Does it matter how happiness is measured? Evidence from a randomized controlled experiment.* Working paper series/Department of Economics 49, University of Zurich. Retrieved February 15, 2016, http://papers.ssrn.com/sol3/papers.cfm?abstract_id=1963817

Valentine, N., Verdes-Tennant, & Bonsel, G. (2015). Health systems' responsiveness and reporting behaviour: Multilevel analysis of the influence of individual-level factors in 64 countries. *Social Science & Medicine, 138*, 152–160.

Veenhoven, R., & Hermus, P. (2006). *Scale interval recorder. Tool for assessing relative weights of verbal response options on survey questions, web survey program.* The Netherlands: Erasmus University Rotterdam, Department of Social Sciences & Risbo Contract Research. http://worlddatabaseofhappiness.eur.nl/images/demo_intervalrecorder.gif

Veenhoven, R. (2008). The international scale interval study. In V. Møller & D. Huschka (Eds.), *Quality of Life in the new millennium: ;Advances in quality-of-life studies, theory and research', Part 2: Refining concepts and measurement to assess cross-cultural quality-of-life, Social Indicator Research Series* (Vol. 35, pp. 45–58). Dordrecht: Springer Press.

Chapter 3
Use of Happiness Scale Interval Studies in This Book

Research Questions Addressed in This Book Using HSIS-Results

In this book we use HSIS-results to address the following research questions.

- Can response scales which appear to be equivalent also be considered to be equivalent when interpreting and mutually comparing survey results? We will go into this question in Chap. 4.
- The overarching question of Chap. 5 is: Is 'Very happy' always equally happy? We have worked this out in three sub-questions:

1. To what extent does the context of the scale affect the evaluation of a given label such as 'Very happy' for a given leading question? This is discussed in section "Evaluation of the labels of response options in the context of the scale".
2. Are the response options of the same item in different languages interpreted differently? This is discussed in section "Interpretation of response options of the same item in different languages".
3. Are the response options of items which only differ in the leading question interpreted differently? This is discussed in section "Different questions about the same topic, but with identical response options".

- Is there a relation between the labeling of anchor points and the assignment of zero-width intervals to response options by judges? This is discussed in Chap. 6.

In this chapter we discuss how the survey items we used to address the research questions were selected and the recruitment process to pick the judges for the studies in which these items were included.

T. de Jonge et al., *Diversity in Survey Questions on the Same Topic*, Social Indicators Research Series 68, DOI 10.1007/978-3-319-53261-5_3

HSIS-Studies Used and the Selection of Survey Items

We have used the results from HSIS-studies conducted in The USA, The Netherlands and Spain to address the research questions formulated above. We will give a short description of each of these studies.

The USA

The University of Notre Dame in Indiana conducted a large HSIS-study in 2014. This study covered a total of forty survey items, equally distributed on the sub-studies English9, English10, English11 and English12. Most of the items were taken from past and recent national surveys fielded in the USA in the last five decades. Some of the items were taken from surveys which were not done in the USA, for purposes of international comparison, for example the Eurobarometer item on life satisfaction we introduced in section "Three scale transformation methods applied to empirical data". The sub-studies English9 and English12 contained only items on happiness. The items in the sub-studies English10 and English11 were restricted to only items on life satisfaction. The division over four studies was mainly done to prevent having too many questions to judge within one study. The sub-studies can therefore essentially be seen to be part of the same study for the purpose of the analyses.

A total of almost 1,100 students were recruited as judges for the study. These judges were split into four groups, each of which participated in one of the sub-studies. This resulted in 348 participants in English9, 270 in English10, 245 in English11 and 233 in English12.

The Netherlands

Statistics Netherlands and the Erasmus University Rotterdam conducted a HSIS-study in 2010 which covered a total of 20 survey items which were equally distributed over the sub-studies Dutch6 and Dutch7. For the same reason as noted for the USA-study, these sub-studies can be considered as one study for the purpose of the analyses. Eighteen of the 20 items in the study were taken from past and recent national surveys fielded in The Netherlands. Two additional items were included aimed at addressing the first of the research questions formulated in section "Research questions addressed in this book using HSIS-results". The first of these additional items was based on an item on life satisfaction included in the study, but with the keyword 'satisfied' replaced by the keyword 'happiness'. Similarly, the second additional item was based on an item on happiness in the study, but with the keyword 'happiness' replaced by the keyword 'satisfied'. The addition of these two extra items, guaranteed that at least two pairs of items in the study meet the conditions for the comparison of survey results, see section "The problem" of Chap. 4. A third pair which met these conditions was found among the other sixteen items included in the study.

The judges for the Dutch HSIS-study were recruited from among students of the Erasmus University Rotterdam and from employees of Statistics Netherlands (CBS) and employees of the Netherlands Institute for Social Research (SCP). Those employed by CBS and SCP could participate in both the sub-studies Dutch6 and Dutch7, however, the students were divided over the two sub-studies. As a result the number of participants in each sub-study was rather large: amounting to 392 judges, 188 employees and 204 students, for Dutch6 and 359 judges: 175 employees and 184 students, for Dutch7.

Spain

The University of Granada set up the HSIS-study Spanish9 which was conducted in two rounds, the first in 2009 and the second a year later in 2010. The study covered a total of ten survey items on happiness and life satisfaction. Although the Spanish study was not set up with the research question of Chap. 4 in mind, the study contained two pairs of items meeting the conditions of section "The problem" of Chap. 4. One of these pairs of items was equivalent to the first pair included in the Dutch study.

The judges for the Spanish study were recruited from among students of the University of Granada, for the first round 198 students were recruited and for the second round 229, amounting to 427 judges in total.

Note: an overview of the wording of the items in Dutch/Spanish and their English equivalents is given in Tables A.1 and A.2 of Appendix A. In these appendices we denoted which of the items are used in Chap. 4. A list of the items used in the study conducted in the USA, for which no translation of the wording was needed is given in Tables B.4–B.7 of Appendix B.

Representativeness of Judges

Items from HSIS-studies are in general assessed by students recruited from the university which conducts the study. An objection to their employment as research participants in social science research is that it is doubtful whether they are representative of the general population because they are on average younger, better educated, to tertiary level, and generally come from more privileged backgrounds than most people in their respective populations (Cummins 2003). Part of the judges in the Dutch HSIS-study consists of non-students, being the judges recruited among employees of Statistics Netherlands and employees of the

Netherlands Institute for Social Research. These employees are probably also not representative of the general population, but they at least represent a different group than that of the judges recruited from the students. The average difference in age between students and employees lies between 20 and 30 years. Furthermore, in contrast to the students, most of the employees have a rather long work experience. We will compare the outcomes for these two groups in the analyses described in Chap. 4, and take advantage of the fact that the HSIS-study in Spain was conducted in two rounds. This allows us to compare the outcomes for these 2 years and those for the pairs of items described in Chap. 4.

A Happiness Scale Interval Study is required employing a group of judges that represents the general population to ascertain that the outcomes are fully valid for the general population, although this may be difficult to organize and is not considered for this book. We want to stress that the Scale Interval Recorder is an instrument that can be used to assess how people interpret words in a common language. We believe that how groups of people evaluate their own happiness may, on average, differ from that in the general population, but that more or less homogeneous groups do not differ substantially in the meanings they assign to words in a common language.

The main statistics of the assessments by students from the HSIS-studies conducted in The Netherlands, Spain and the USA are reported in Appendix B and consist for each item of the number of valid assessments, for the assessment of the upper boundary of each response option, (1) the mean value, (2) the standard deviation and (3) the standard error and for the anchor points of each response scale the number of judges who assigned a zero-width interval to the corresponding response options by choosing the upper and lower bound both equal to an extreme of the continuum (Kalmijn 2010, p. 147 sqq).

References

Cummins, R. A. (2003). Normative life satisfaction: Measurement issues and homeostatic model. *Social Indicators Research, 64*, 225–240.

Kalmijn, W. M. (2010). *Quantification of happiness inequality*. Dissertation, Erasmus University Rotterdam, The Netherlands. Enschede: Ipskamp Drukkers. Available at http://repub.eur.nl/pub/21777

Chapter 4
Equivalence of Rating Scales Using Different Keywords

Surveys with Equivalent Items for 'Happiness' and 'Satisfaction with Life'

To determine whether or not equivalent response options for happiness and satisfaction with life are interpreted equivalently, an obvious step is to measure both topics in one survey and to compare the response patterns. The comparability of such a study however, largely depends on the variations in survey items of which a difference in the keywords used is just one. Each variation will influence the response patterns and therefore an approach to verify that a difference in response patterns has to be attributed to the differences in keywords used, needs to exclude other variations in the items. In the case of happiness and life satisfaction, this would require a study that includes items for both topics which have equivalent response scales and only differ in the keyword used. The method we present in this book focuses on response scales with verbal labels for all response options and thus excludes response scales with no verbal labels or only verbally labeled anchor points. In the collection 'Measures of Happiness' of the WDH only a few studies can be found that meet both these requirements. These eighteen studies are presented in Table 4.1.

The means of the ratings for happiness and life satisfaction have been reported in all the 18 studies. In 14 out of the 18 pairs people rate their happiness higher than their satisfaction with life. In half of the cases, all from the studies done by the Leisure Development Centre (1980), the difference in reported means for happiness and life satisfaction was less than 0.1 point.[1] The largest of the eighteen reported differences is found in the study done by Michalos and Orlando (2006) and is equal to 0.3 points. In the WDH gamma correlations between happiness and satisfaction

[1]We are aware that if the means for happiness and life satisfaction are equal, it does not necessarily imply that the constructs for both topics measure the same and that the correlation between the two topics can still be low.

T. de Jonge et al., *Diversity in Survey Questions on the Same Topic*, Social Indicators Research Series 68, DOI 10.1007/978-3-319-53261-5_4

Table 4.1 Survey studies that involve questions on both 'happiness' and 'life satisfaction'

The Leisure Development Centre (1980) (13 studies)		Ventegodt (1996) (1 study)	
How happy do you feel as you live now? Please choose one item on this card that comes closest to your feeling.	Overall, how satisfied are you with your present life?	How happy are you now?	How satisfied are you with your life now?
1. Very unhappy	1. Very dissatisfied	1. Very unhappy	1. Very dissatisfied
2. Fairly unhappy	2. Fairly dissatisfied	2. Fairly unhappy	2. Fairly dissatisfied
3. Neither happy nor unhappy	3. Neither satisfied nor dissatisfied	3. Neither happy nor unhappy	4. Fairly satisfied
4. Fairly happy	4, Fairly satisfied	4. Fairly happy	4. Fairly satisfied
5. Very happy	5. Very satisfied	5. Very happy	5. Very satisfied
Michalos and Zumbo (1999, 2003); Michalos (2003); Michalos and Orlando (2006) (4 studies)			
Considering your life as a whole, how happy would you say you are?		How satisfied are you with your life as a whole?	
1. Very unhappy		1. Very dissatisfied	
2. Somewhat unhappy		2. Somewhat dissatisfied	
3. A little unhappy		3. A little dissatisfied	
4. About evenly balanced		4. About evenly balanced	
5. A little happy		5. A little satisfied	
6. Somewhat happy		6. Somewhat satisfied	
7. Very happy		7. Very satisfied	

Source: World Database of Happiness, collection Measures of Happiness (Veenhoven 2016)

with life have been calculated for all the studies of the Leisure Development Centre (LDC). These gamma correlations fluctuate between 0.62 and 0.88. Michalos and Orlando (2006) and Ventegodt (1996) report Pearson correlation coefficients for the relationship between happiness and life satisfaction of 0.73 and 0.72 respectively. There is no clear relationship between these correlation coefficients and the differences between the means of happiness and life satisfaction.

In most of the studies listed in Table 4.1, happiness and life satisfaction are related to satisfaction with a number of life domains, such as family, social relations, income, education, health, politics, et cetera, using equivalent response scales. Although some studies show a small difference between mean happiness and mean satisfaction with life, both topics may have a rather different relation to satisfaction with one of those life domains: in France for example, the differences in means between happiness and life satisfaction in the study of the Leisure Development Centre was only 0.02. The gamma correlation between happiness and the level of education however, was 0.21, whereas the gamma correlation of this life domain with satisfaction with life was no higher than 0.04.

The Problem

The discussion presented in the previous section gives rise to the question: Can response scales which appear to be equivalent also be considered to be equivalent when interpreting and mutually comparing survey results?

The means and correlations, discussed in section "Surveys with equivalent items for 'happiness' and 'satisfaction with life'" are, according to common practice, all based on the ranks of the response options, disregarding the interval on a 0–10 continuum corresponding to each response option. In this common practice it is implicitly assumed that equivalent response options in equivalent scales on different topics are valued equivalently. Yet, this may contradict reality, as it brings with it the risk of muddling the results when comparing survey outcomes due to differences in the interpretation of each scale by the respondents. Therefore, to prevent this risk occurring, this difference in interpretation must be examined and discussed carefully beforehand. Although in recent research this problem had been addressed (e.g. Saris and Gallhofer 2007, 2014, Ch. 16), we focus on a new method that is suitable to dealing with such an examination in this chapter.

The Scale Interval Recorder as an Instrument to Compare the Intervals Represented by Equivalent Response Options

The Scale Interval Recorder was initially developed to compare the interval corresponding to, identical or non-identical, response options in different response scales on the *same* topic, for example happiness or life satisfaction. The instrument however, can also be used to investigate whether equivalent response options in equivalent scales that only differ in the keywords used, represent an equal interval. For this purpose, we require that a pair of survey items meets the following conditions:

- the question of each item must correspond to the topic, in this book happiness or satisfaction with life, used for the labels of the response options
- the questions posed in both items must refer to the same time frame, for example life as a whole, the past 4 weeks or at this moment
- the response scales of both items must be equivalent, having the same number of response options, which by themselves may only differ in the topic they refer to

Once one or more pairs of items that fulfill these conditions have been selected, the Scale Interval Recorder can be used for a group of judges to assess the response scales of these items.

We will explain the method for testing the equivalence of rating scales using different keywords, which we described in section "The problem" of Chap. 4, using a mutual comparison of the assessment of the scales of three pairs of items presented in the Dutch HSIS-study, two pairs of items assessed by Spanish judges and five pairs of items from the HSIS-study conducted in the USA. As we remarked in section "Representativeness of judges" we also make use of the opportunity, to split the assessments for the items from the Dutch study into those by students and those by employees. The assessments for the items from the Spanish studies are split into those of 2009 and those of 2010.

We first consider the Dutch questions and compare both level and dispersion of the assessments of the boundaries between the response options for the students and the employees. Next we do the same for the 2 years of Spanish assessments and for the results of the USA study.

Differences in Value Ranges Represented by Response Options Labeled in Dutch, Spanish and English

Response Options Labeled in Dutch

The first pair of items from the Dutch HSIS-study consists of an item on happiness taken from the World Values Survey (WVS) and an item on life satisfaction from the Eurobarometer. Both items have a 4-point symmetric response scale, without an explicit neutral midpoint. The assessments of the response options in the scales, given by Dutch judges are depicted in Fig. 4.1, juxtaposing the average assessments for the response options for happiness and life satisfaction for the students and the employees.

From a quick visual inspection of Fig. 4.1, we can conclude that the students and the employees evaluate the response options of the item on happiness equally to those of the item on life satisfaction. There are however, some minor differences between the assessments by the students and the employees. The biggest difference between the two groups of judges is present for the response options beginning with 'Fairly'. The length of the interval assigned to these options by the employees is on average 0.3 points smaller, than the interval assigned by the students.

The average assessments and the standard errors of their estimated mean values of the upper boundaries for the pair of items depicted in Fig. 4.1 are given in Table 4.2. In the left column of Table 4.2 only the adverbs used in the wording of each response option is given. The averages in Table 4.2, in combination with the small standard errors, underpin the conclusion that Dutch judges on average evaluate the scales for happiness and satisfaction with life from pair 1 equally.

As we mentioned in section "HSIS-studies used and the selection of survey items", two items in the Dutch HSIS-study are variations on other items in the available Dutch survey data with happiness or life satisfaction being used equivalent. In the study list of the WDH, these two items for the purpose of answering the research question formulated in section "The scale interval recorder as an instrument to compare the intervals represented by equivalent response options" are referred to as experimental. The first of the variations is an item on happiness and

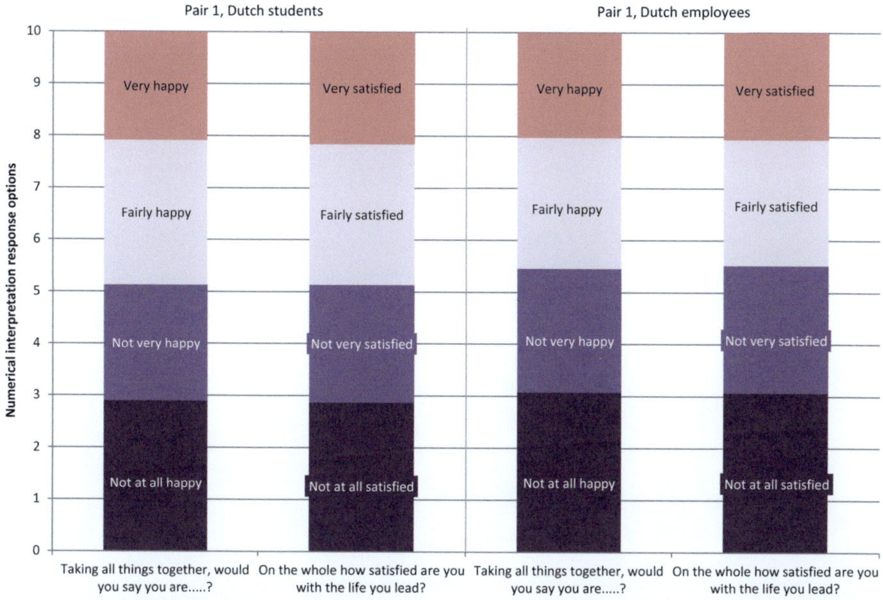

Fig. 4.1 Comparison of the interpretation of verbal response scales by Dutch students and employees

Table 4.2 Average and standard error assessment of upper boundaries by Dutch judges

	Pair 1, Dutch students				Pair 1, Dutch employees			
	Happiness		Satisfaction		Happiness		Satisfaction	
Abbrev. response option	Average	Std. err	Average	Std. err	Average	Std. err	Average	Std. err
Very	10.0	–	10.0	–	10.0	–	10.0	–
Fairly	7.9	0.07	7.8	0.06	8.0	0.07	7.9	0.06
Not very	5.1	0.09	5.1	0.09	5.5	0.07	5.5	0.07
Not at all	2.9	0.11	2.9	0.11	3.1	0.10	3.1	0.10

is treated as equivalent to the item on life satisfaction, introduced earlier, which was taken from a Statistics Netherlands (CBS) survey. In a similar manner, an item on life satisfaction has been created which is treated as equivalent to a 5-point scale item on happiness taken from the Dutch Household Survey (DHS). With these two experimental items we have made sure that we have two pairs of items that meet the conditions formulated in section "The scale interval recorder as an instrument to compare the intervals represented by equivalent response options".

The second and third pair of items, depicted in Fig. 4.2, are identical in the leading questions for happiness and life satisfaction, but have rather different response scales. The response scales of the items forming the second pair are symmetric and have a neutral midpoint. We have discussed the asymmetry of the response scales of the items comprising the third pair of items in section "An

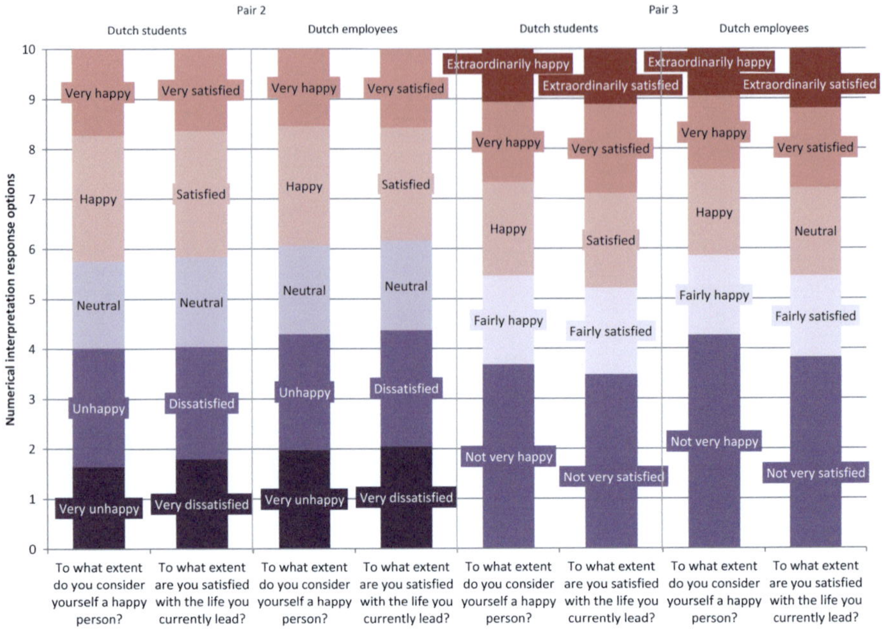

Fig. 4.2 Comparison of the interpretation of verbal response scales by Dutch students and employees

impression of the diversity in survey items". The assessments of the response options from the scales of the second and third pair by the students and the employees are depicted in Fig. 4.2.

As for the first pair of items, for the second pair of items the intervals assigned to the response options for happiness are equal in most cases to those for the life satisfaction options for the second pair of items. This can be noticed for both students and employees. There is a slight difference in evaluation of the response options between the students and the employees, the biggest difference between the two groups of judges is seen for the response option 'Very unhappy', to which the employees assign an interval that is on average 0.6 point longer than the interval assigned by the students. This difference is by far the largest we found in the Dutch HSIS-study (DeJonge et al. 2015, pp. 98–100).

Unlike for the first and second pair of items taken from the Dutch HSIS-study, the response options for happiness for the third pair of items were assessed differently from those for life satisfaction by the students and the employees, and, again, the assessment of the employees differs from that of the students. Yet, the differences in the assessment of the response options for happiness, compared to life satisfaction, go into the same direction for the students and the employees.

Although for the third pair of items from the Dutch HSIS-study there are differences between happiness and life satisfaction in the evaluation of the response options, these differences are small when compared to the differences in intervals of

Table 4.3 Average and standard error assessment of upper boundaries by Dutch judges

	Pair 2, Dutch students				Pair 2, Dutch employees			
	Happiness		Satisfaction		Happiness		Satisfaction	
Abbrev. response option	Average	Std. err	Average	Std. err	Average	Std. err	Average	Std. err
Very h/s	10.0	–	10.0	–	10.0	–	10.0	–
Hap/Sat	8.3	0.05	8.4	0.06	8.5	0.05	8.4	0.05
Neutral	5.8	0.08	5.8	0.07	6.1	0.06	6.2	0.05
Un/Dis	4.0	0.09	4.0	0.08	4.3	0.08	4.4	0.07
Very u/d	1.6	0.07	1.8	0.08	2.0	0.08	2.0	0.08
	Pair 3, Dutch students				Pair 3, Dutch employees			
	Happiness		Satisfaction		Happiness		Satisfaction	
Abbrev. response option	Average	Std. err	Average	Std. err	Average	Std. err	Average	Std. err
Extraord.	10.0	–	10.0	–	10.0	–	10.0	–
Very	8.9	0.06	8.9	0.05	9.1	0.06	8.8	0.06
Hap/Sat	7.3	0.07	7.1	0.07	7.6	0.07	7.2	0.09
Fairly	5.5	0.11	5.2	0.10	5.9	0.09	5.5	0.11
Not very	3.7	0.14	3.5	0.13	4.3	0.12	3.8	0.13

similar response options in dissimilar scales. For example the response option 'Fairly satisfied' in the 4-point scale of the first pair is evaluated very differently compared to the same option in the 5-point scale of the third pair. In other words, the meaning given by respondents to the labels of response options is not fixed, but depends on the number of options given to choose from and the labels attached to the options. The average assessments and the standard errors of their estimated mean values for the upper boundaries of the pairs of items depicted in Fig. 4.2 are given in Table 4.3 using abbreviations of the wording of the response options.

The standard errors of the assessments of the upper boundaries of the response options in the lower part of the scales of the third pair of items are remarkably large compared to those found for the other pairs of items. It is likely that this is induced by the asymmetry of the scales of the items in the third pair, which might also explain in part the difference in the outcomes of the assessments between students and employees. Although the assessments of the students and the employees point in the same direction, we will only use the assessments made by the Dutch students to support of this discussion, since the judges from Spain and the USA are also students.

Response Options Labeled in Spanish

There are two pairs of items available from the Spanish HSIS-study, which were assessed by different groups of students in 2009 and in 2010. An item on happiness taken from the Eurobarometer and an item on life satisfaction taken from the International Tension Study make up the first pair. The second pair consists of an item on happiness taken from the World Values Survey (WVS) and an item on life satisfaction taken from the Latino Barometer. The assessments of the response options to the scales of these items by the Spanish judges are depicted in Fig. 4.3. The translation from Spanish into English of the leading questions for both pairs of items is the same, but from Table A.2 appendix A it can be seen that these questions are different, although we consider them as equivalent. The second pair in Fig. 4.3 is equivalent to pair 1, presented in Fig. 4.1, assessed by the Dutch judges. The difference between these two pairs is in the item for life satisfaction. The question in the Spanish version of the life satisfaction item in pair 1 in Fig. 4.1 is "En general, ¿qué tan satisfecho está con el tipo de vida que lleva?" which can be considered as equivalent to the life satisfaction question of the item in pair 1 in Fig. 4.3 which is formulated as "En términos generales, ¿diría Ud. que está satisfecho/a con su vida?". The problem however, is entailed in the labeling of the response options. Instead of 'Bastante satisfecho/a', as is used for one of the response options of the item in Fig. 4.3, the label for the item in Fig. 4.1 used in the Spanish studies is 'Más bien satisfecho'. The difference between 'bastante' and 'más bien' is too large to consider these labels as equivalent, also because these labels are attached to response options which are not at the end of the scale. Therefore we had to turn to the item for life satisfaction presented in Fig. 4.3. One could argue that 'nada' and

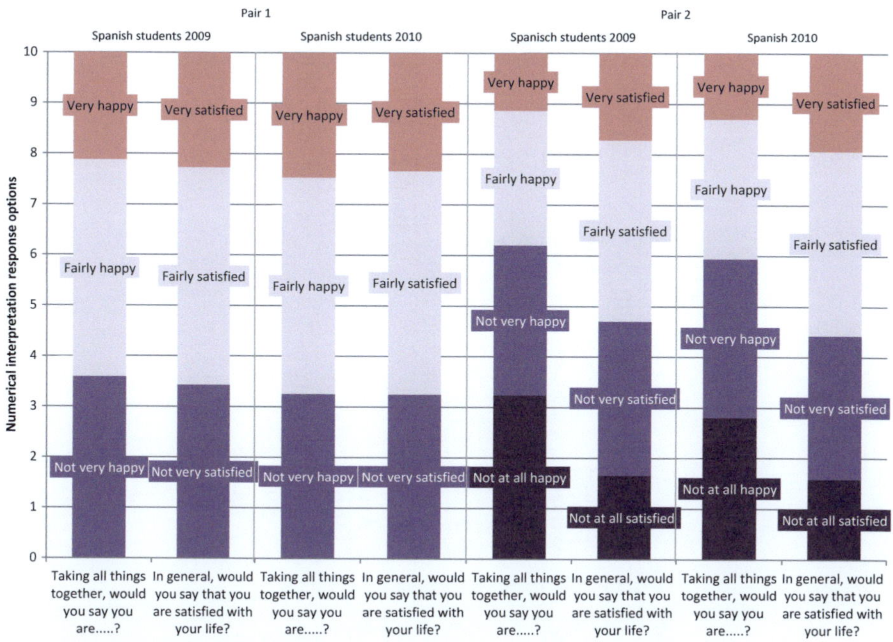

Fig. 4.3 Comparison of the interpretation of verbal response scales by Spanish students

'para nada' are also not fully equivalent, but since these words in the labels of the response options are at the lower end of the scale, this is, in view of the small observed frequencies, of minor importance.

The judges from Spain interpreted the response options of the 3-point scale items almost identically, but the intervals in 2009 differ slightly from those in 2010. There was more visible difference in the assessments by the Dutch judges; however, noticeable differences can be observed in the interpretations by the Spanish judges in their assessments of the 4-point scales. The difference in interpretation between 2009 and 2010 by the Spanish judges is also small for the 4-point scales. Given the results shown in Fig. 4.3, the impression is that Spanish people more easily rate themselves as being satisfied with life than as being happy, in the sense that for pair 2 the bar for being happy is set higher than for being satisfied. In both Spanish pairs, the value range assigned to the response options at the lower end of the scale is higher for life satisfaction than for happiness.

It can be seen from Table 4.4 that the standard errors of the estimated mean values of the assessments of the upper boundaries of the response options of the items from the Spanish HSIS-study are reasonably small. From that we conclude that the Spanish judges in general evaluate the scales for happiness and satisfaction with life differently.

Since we did not find any relevant differences between the assessments of 2009 and 2010, we combined the assessments for the remainder of the discussion.

Table 4.4 Average and standard error assessment of upper boundaries by Spanish judges

	Pair 1, Spanish students 2009				Pair 1, Spanish students 2010			
	Happiness		Satisfaction		Happiness		Satisfaction	
Abbrev. response option	Average	Std. err	Average	Std. err	Average	Std. err	Average	Std. err
Very h/s	10.0	–	10.0	–	10.0	–	10.0	–
Fairly	7.9	0.12	7.7	0.11	7.5	0.10	7.7	0.11
Not very	3.6	0.14	3.4	0.15	3.2	0.13	3.2	0.15
	Pair 2, Spanish students 2009				Pair 2, Spanish students 2010			
	Happiness		Satisfaction		Happiness		Satisfaction	
Abbrev. response option	Average	Std. err	Average	Std. err	Average	Std. err	Average	Std. err
Very	10.0	–	10.0	–	10.0	–	10.0	–
Fairly	8.9	0.10	8.3	0.05	8.7	0.08	8.1	0.09
Not very	6.2	0.12	4.7	0.07	5.9	0.12	4.4	0.12
Not at all	3.2	0.15	1.7	0.10	2.8	0.14	1.6	0.10

Response Options Labeled in English

Among the items from the HSIS-study done in the USA, we have found three pairs of items using 4-point scales and two pairs of items using 5-points scales, which meet the requirements from section "The scale interval recorder as an instrument to compare the intervals represented by equivalent response options". The first 4-point scale pair consists of an item on happiness taken from the Gallup World Survey and the same item on life satisfaction from the Eurobarometer which was part of the first pair from the Dutch HSIS-study. The items from the second 4-point scale pair were both taken from the USA Gallup Polls and the items from the third pair were both taken from the Canadian General Social Survey. A 5-point scale item on happiness taken from the South African Periodical Quality of Life Survey and a 5-point scale item on life satisfaction taken from the New Zealand General Social Survey make up the fourth pair. The fifth pair consists of 5-point scale items from the survey of the Leisure Development Centre (LDC) which we presented in Table 4.1 and an additional item on life satisfaction which in our opinion is also equivalent to the item on happiness in this fifth pair. The assessments of the response options for the 4-point scale items by American judges are depicted in Fig. 4.4.

We conclude from a visual inspection of Fig. 4.4, that the American judges evaluate the response options of the items on happiness equally to those of the items on life satisfaction. The difference in the lengths of the intervals for equivalent response options is in all cases less than 0.1. This also holds for the differences in intervals between the items of different pairs with identical response scales, we will discuss further in section "Different questions about the same topic, but with identical response options". The standard errors of the estimated mean values of the assessments of the upper boundaries of the response options of the items from Fig. 4.4 are given in Table 4.5.

The averages of the boundaries in Table 4.5, in combination with the small standard errors, support the conclusion that American judges on average evaluate the 4-point scales for happiness and satisfaction with life equally. This is comparable to the results we found for the first pair of items taken from the Dutch HSIS-study.

The results for the pairs of items with 5-point scales in the American HSIS-study are remarkable as becomes clear from a look at Fig. 4.5.

Looking at the assessments of the fourth pair, we get the same impression as for the pairs depicted in Fig. 4.4 for the American HSIS-study. This is also the case for the fifth pair of the study if we compare the item on happiness with the additional item on life satisfaction. If we, however, compare the item on happiness from this pair with the item on life satisfaction from the same survey of the LDC, than we have to conclude that the scale are interpreted differently. An explanation for this can probably found in the differences in leading question which we will discuss in section "Different questions about the same topic, but with identical response options". Given the research question as formulated in section "The problem" of this chapter, we conclude that the comparability of the results for happiness and life

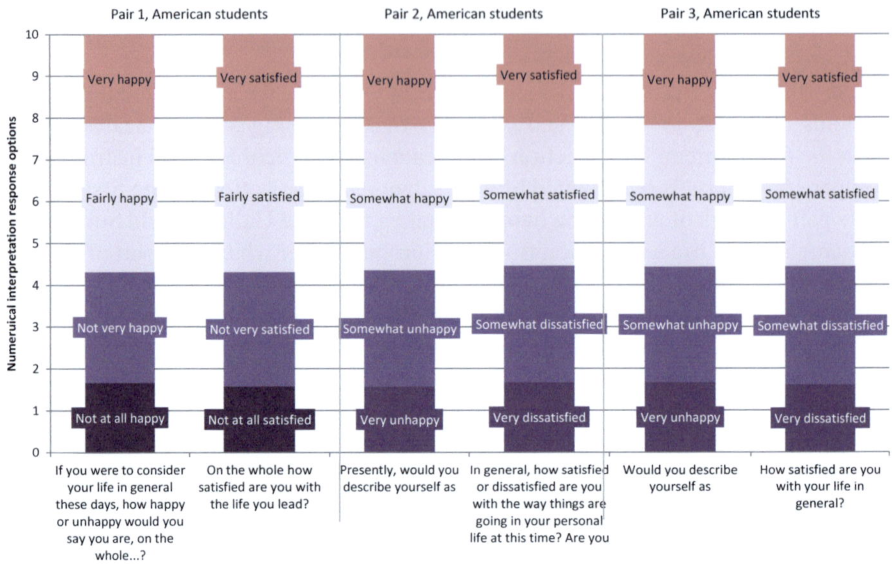

Fig. 4.4 Comparison of the interpretation of verbal response scales by American students

Table 4.5 Average and standard error assessment of upper boundaries by American judges

	Pair 1, American students			
	Happiness		Satisfaction	
Abbrev. response option	Average	Std. err	Average	Std. err
Very	10.0	–	10.0	–
Fairly	7.9	0.06	7.9	0.07
Not very	4.3	0.08	4.3	0.09
Not at all	1.7	0.07	1.6	0.08
	Pair 2, American students			
	Happiness		Satisfaction	
Abbrev. response option	Average	Std. err	Average	Std. err
Very	10.0	–	10.0	–
Fairly	7.8	0.07	7.9	0.07
Not very	4.4	0.08	4.5	0.08
Not at all	1.6	0.07	1.7	0.07
	Pair 3, American students			
	Happiness		Satisfaction	
Abbrev. response option	Average	Std. err	Average	Std. err
Very	10.0	–	10.0	–
Fairly	7.8	0.07	7.9	0.08
Not very	4.4	0.09	4.4	0.09
Not at all	1.7	0.08	1.6	0.07

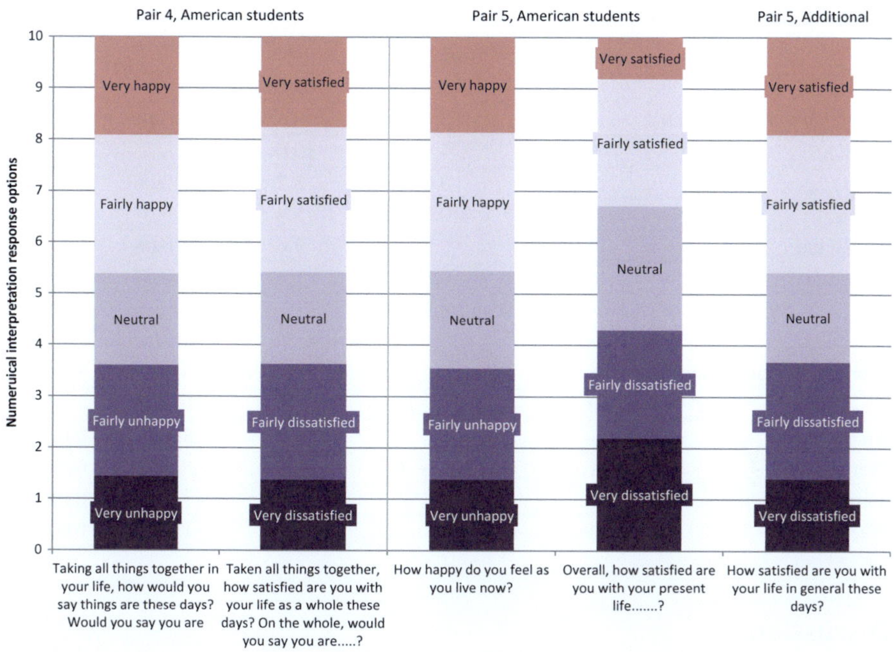

Fig. 4.5 Comparison of the interpretation of verbal response scales by American students

satisfaction from the survey of the LDC is probably comprised by a difference in the interpretations of the response scales. We will illustrate this using the frequency distributions for happiness and life satisfaction in the LDC survey done in the USA in 1979 which are equal to respectively {0.9%, 2.4%, 7.0%, 47.9%, 41.7%} and {1.3%, 3.9%, 6.1%, 51.4%, 37.1%} ordered in ascending order of the ranks of the response options. Using the Rank Method, see section "The incomparability of time series from different surveys and different time periods", these frequency distributions would result in a mean value of 4.27 for happiness and a marginally lower mean value of 4.19 for life satisfaction. While using the Weighted Average Approach and the mid-interval values of the intervals shown in Fig. 4.5, the mean value for happiness would be equal to 7.42 and be exceeded notably by the mean value for life satisfaction of 8.12. We will not comment upon which of the two differences is most reliable, the one using the Rank Method or that using the Weighted Average Approach, but want to stress that the results point in different directions.

The means and standard errors of the assessments for the 5-point scales pairs of items from the American HSIS-study are Table 4.6.

Table 4.6 Average and standard error assessment of upper boundaries by American judges

	Pair 4, American students			
	Happiness		Satisfaction	
Abbrev. response option	Average	Std. err	Average	Std. err
Very h/s	10.0	–	10.0	–
Fairly h/s	8.1	0.06	8.2	0.06
Neutral	5.4	0.07	5.4	0.07
Fairly u/d	3.6	0.07	3.6	0.08
Very u/d	1.4	0.07	1.4	0.07

	Pair 5, American students					
	Happiness		Satisfaction		Satisfaction (altern.)	
Abbrev. response option	Average	Std. err	Average	Std. err	Average	Std. err
Very h/s	10.0	–	10.0	–	10.0	–
Fairly h/s	8.1	0.05	9.2	0.07	8.1	0.07
Neutral	5.4	0.06	6.7	0.08	5.4	0.08
Fairly u/d	3.5	0.06	4.3	0.09	3.7	0.08
Very u/d	1.4	0.05	2.2	0.10	1.4	0.07

Discussion

Methodological Consideration

Current and past practices show that in many studies in which topics such as happiness and satisfaction with life are related to other aspects of life, the scales of the items that are associated are dissimilar. In order to be convinced that results will not be compromised due to the incomparability of the scales or differences in the interpretation of each scale by the respondents, in future research the scales of items that will be compared, have to be examined and discussed carefully and equivalent agreed on before any comparisons are made. The Scale Interval Recorder is a useful instrument to do this since it offers the opportunity to have the response scales that are used in a study assessed by judges and this to get an indication whether these scales might be interpreted differently or not by different judges.

Limitations

The results presented in this book for the interpretation of survey items by native Dutch, Spanish and English speaking judges are based on a limited number of pairs of items on happiness and satisfaction with life and cannot be said to represent the large variation found in survey items. The conclusions drawn are only valid for the type of items that can, and have been, mutually compared. To generalize these findings further research is needed to investigate the equivalence of scales for extended sets of pairs of survey items that to get results better represents the large variation in survey items.

Implication of the Method

When searching for pairs of items with equivalent response options for happiness and life satisfaction we found that the occurrence of equivalency in one language does not mean that this equivalency will also exists for a corresponding pair labeled in another language. This was a by-product of our research, one from which we could conclude that the translation of the labels of response options may come with, what we call, a translation bias that reduces the comparability of survey responses between language groups.

Advice for Further Research

If only one pair of items has to be assessed, it is likely that the assessment of the scale of the second item will be influenced by the assessment of the scale of the first item, if they are presented successively to the judges. An option to prevent this form of bias is to split the group of judges into two equally representative groups and to have each group assess one of the items or both items but present them in reverse order to the groups. Another option is to include the pair of items in a series of items that are part of a Scale Interval Study as was the case for the pairs of items used in the example we present in this book.

If more pairs of items have to be assessed, it seems to make sense for the same reason as mentioned in the previous point, to split the group of judges in two and to have each group assess one item of each pair. If the group of judges is split to have each group assess one item of each pair, another choice is to have each group assess only the items on the same topic or items for both topics.

Conclusion

Equivalent response scales do not always elicit well comparable responses across topics, population subgroups and languages. Comparative analysis requires therefore that comparability of response scales is assessed in advance. The Scale Interval Recorder can be used for that purpose.

References

DeJonge, T., Veenhoven, R., & Arends, L. R. (2015). 'Very Happy' is not always equally happy on the meaning of verbal response options in survey questions. *Journal of Happiness Studies, 16* (1), 77–101. doi:10.1007/s10902-013-9497-9.

Michalos, A. C. (2003). Policing services and the quality of life. *Social Indicators Research, 61*, 1–18. doi:10.1023/A:1021259917948.

Michalos, A. C., & Orlando, J. A. (2006). A note on student quality of life. *Social Indicators Research, 79*, 51–59. doi:10.1007/s11205-005-2404-y.

Michalos, A. C., & Zumbo, B. D. (1999). Public services and the quality of life. *Social Indicators Research, 48*, 125–156. doi:10.1023/A:1006893225196.

Michalos, A. C., & Zumbo, B. D. (2003). Leisure activities, health and the quality of life. In A. C. Michalos (Ed.), *Essays on the quality of life* (pp. 217–238). Dordrecht: Kluwer.

Saris, W. E., & Gallhofer, I. N. (2007). *Design, evaluation, and analysis of questionnaires for survey research* (Wiley series in survey methodology). New York: Wiley-Interscience. ISBN 978-0-470-11495-7, e-ISBN 978–0–470-16519-5.

Saris, W. E., & Gallhofer, I. N. (2014). *Design, evaluation, and analysis of questionnaires for survey research* (Wiley series in survey methodology, 2nd ed.). New York: Wiley-Interscience. ISBN 978-0-470-11495-7, ISBN 978–1–118-63461-5.

The Leisure Development Center. (1980). *Survey of values in 13 countries. Table book for the 1980 international conference on human values.* Tokyo: The Leisure Development Center. http://worlddatabaseofhappiness.eur.nl/hap_bib/freetexts/~LeisureDevelopmentCentre_1980.pdf. Accessed 29 Jan 2016.

Veenhoven, R. (2016). *Measures of Happiness. World Database of happiness.* Rotterdam: Erasmus University Rotterdam. Available at: http://worlddatabaseofhappiness.eur.nl/hap_quer/hqi_fp.htm

Ventegodt, S. (1996). *Liskvalitet hos 4500 31-33-arige.* (The Quality of Life of 4500 31-33-Years-Olds). Copenhagen: Forskningscentrets Forlag.

Chapter 5
'Very Happy' Is Not Always Equally Happy

Evaluation of the Labels of Response Options in the Context of the Scale

The Semantic Judgment of Fixed Word Value Method Revisited

We gave a brief description of the Semantic Judgment of Fixed Word Value Method in section "Conventional scale transformation methods for items from different surveys". The study of Jones and Thurstone (1955), referred to in that section, stems from the idea that the meaning of a word depends on the context in which it is presented. Jones and Thurstone asked a group of respondents to rate the meaning of 51 words and phrases people use to describe a like or a dislike of a food on a discrete 9-point interval scale from −4 to 4. This resulted in a list of meaning values for all these words and phrases. Jones and Thurstone conclude that the results of their study make it possible to select suitable descriptive adjectives for use as labels for successive intervals on subsequent preference schedules. A method similar to that of Jones and Thurstone was applied by Veenhoven (1993, pp. 109–112) and 12 co-workers to the response options of survey items on happiness and life satisfaction, to obtain comparable average scores. More recently, Braunsberger and Gates (2009) adopted the method of Jones and Thurstone in the field of marketing research for 39 items on satisfaction and 19 Likert[1] items. They conclude that their inventories of mean values and standard deviations for scale point descriptors should be of interest to industry and academia, because knowledge of a scale point descriptor's mean value allows the construction of successive interval or equal interval scales that can be used to support meaningful statistical analyses and interpretation of data.

[1]Likert items are items with response options labeled in terms of agreement.

T. de Jonge et al., *Diversity in Survey Questions on the Same Topic*, Social Indicators Research Series 68, DOI 10.1007/978-3-319-53261-5_5

As Jones and Thurstone (1955, p. 31) remarked, a word has an infinite number of connotations, each corresponding to a particular context and therefore it is not possible to determine, either logically or experimentally the generalized meaning of a word. The result of a Semantic Judgment of Fixed Word Value Method however, is, as noted, a list of meaning values for all labels assessed in the study. In our opinion, these meaning values are of less value if they are used as fixed word values, due to their dependency on the context of the scale. It is more likely that the list should merely be seen as an ordering of appropriate adjectives, which may be useful when, for some kind of reason, one wants to construct a new verbal rating scale. The comparability problem cannot be solved with this method as we have illustrated in Table 2.2.

Research Question In line with the remarks of Jones and Thurstone about the infinite number of meanings a word can have, we formulated the following research question: To what extent does the context of the scale affect the evaluation of a given label such as 'Very happy' for a given leading question?

The Context of the Scale and Comparability

From the results of HSIS-studies, we selected a number of groups of items where the items within a group have been evaluated by judges from the same country, have the same leading question, the same number of response options but are different in the labeling of these options. We selected two groups of three items, one assessed by Dutch judges and one by American judges and three groups of two items, all assessed by American judges. The results for the item groups with three items are presented in Fig. 5.1 and the results for the other groups in Fig. 5.2. The code according to the classification of the WDH is given above each item, as a reference.

The 5-point items assessed by the Dutch students are very informative with respect to the research question. The differences between the first two items of this group are seen in the lower part of the scales. The second item has a symmetric scale, which is more extreme in the lower part than the first items. It can be seen in Fig. 5.1, that the meaning interval, to use Jones and Thurstone's wording, assigned to the label 'Not very happy' of the first item is more or less the same as that assigned to the label 'Unhappy' of the second item. The word 'Unhappy' in this second scale, appears to express something different from the same word in the scale of the first item. The addition of the rather extreme anchor point at the upper part of the third item assessed by the Dutch students turns out to lower the meaning intervals of all the other response options in the scale when compared to the first two items in this group. The item with the label 'Fairly happy' even seems to come with a more or less negative connotation in this scale, whereas the label 'Happy' has taken the place of the neutral option of other items. It is very likely that the answer given by a respondent is influenced by the position of the response option on the

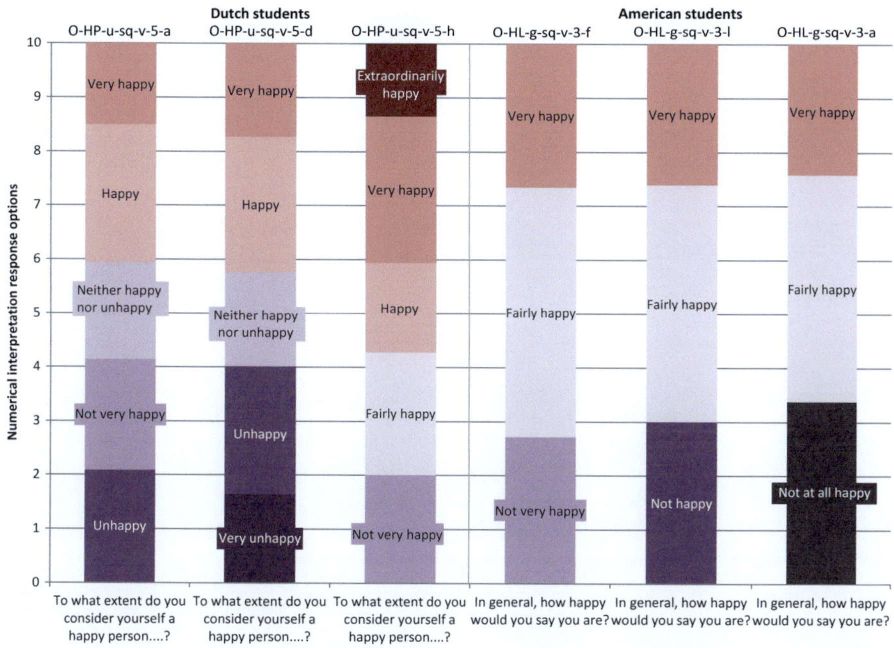

Fig. 5.1 The effect of the context of the scale on the meaning of verbal labels, part 1

scale. Someone who is happy would consider a response option, even if it is labeled 'Happy', in the middle of the scale not in concordance with this, this could tempt these people to choose the option 'Very happy', since this is the position on the scale that is more in harmony with their perception happiness (DeJonge et al. 2015, p. 92).

The items in the three-item group assessed by the American students differ in the label of the lowest response option. According to the value meaning list found by Veenhoven (1993, p. 110) and the list found by Braunsberger and Gates (2009, p. 223), in the latter case about satisfaction in the field of marketing, the value of the phrase 'Not very happy' is higher than that of 'Not happy', which on its turn has a higher value than the phrase 'Not at all happy'. Yet, this value order is not apparent in Fig. 5.1. Given the two value lists mentioned, it would have been more likely, that the length of the interval assigned to the option 'Not at all happy' would be smaller than the lengths of the intervals of the lower options of the two other items in this group. We do not have a conclusive explanation for this.

The results presented in Fig. 5.2 underpin the conclusion which can be drawn from Fig. 5.1 that the meaning assigned to the wording of a response option is to a large extent determined by the context of the scale. The meaning of the wording of a label in one scale, may be taken over by the wording of a neighboring label if this label is attached to a response option with a different position on the scale of another item but with the same leading question.

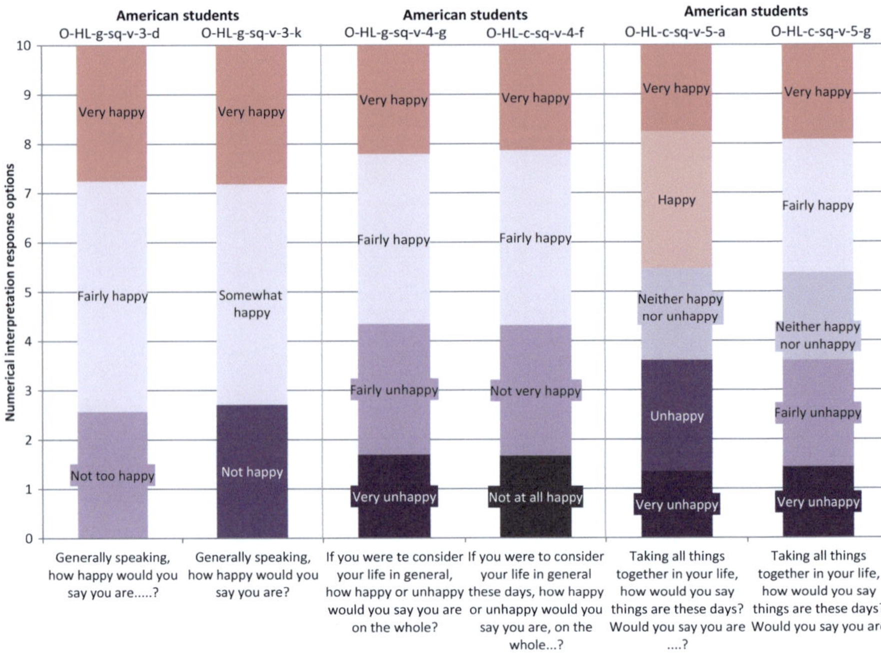

Fig. 5.2 The context of the scale on the meaning of verbal labels, part 2

Interpretation of Response Options of the Same Item in Different Languages

Translation and Comparability

It is necessary that questions depict the intended concepts accurately and that the respondents are familiar with the question's wording in their native language for the comparability of perceptions and opinions of people across countries (Eurofound 2010, p. 2) and, normally for international surveys[2] a strict translation procedure is followed. The translation procedures for the European Social Survey (ESS), for example, are based on a number of key principles, such as that the source questionnaire is designed in British English and then translated item by item by each language team which follows the TRAPD methodology, where TRAPD stands for Translation, Review, Adjudication, Pretesting and Documentation.[3] For the Gallup World Poll, the process includes a source questionnaire in English, two independent translations, back translations and survey personnel who adjudicate the differences

[2]A broad overview of European surveys on opinions and perceptions can be found on the website of the European Data Center for Work and Welfare (EDAC), www.edac.eu

[3]http://www.europeansocialsurvey.org/methodology/translation.html. Assessed 25 March 2015.

(Gallup 2007). To quote Harkness et al. (2010, p. 117), a successful translation is expected 'to keep the content of the questions semantically similar within the bounds of the target language, keep the question format similar; retain measurement properties, including the range of response options offered; and maintain the same stimulus', while McDowell (2006, p. 14) states: 'translation is approached from outside and seeks to derive a non-culture-specific presentation of the underlying ideas, which are assumed to be universally applicable'.

The issue of translation must be considered as yet another dimension of the comparability problem, coming on top of the problems caused by the diversity in survey items as discussed in section "An impression of the diversity in survey items". The issue of translation makes clear that it is not only the differences in interpretation of response options by respondents that have to be accounted for when comparing survey results, we also have to take into account that a difference that might occur in interpretations of response options by translators. This is exemplified by Saris (1997, p. 122) using the response options for the 4-point scale item on life satisfaction taken from the Eurobarometer. He remarks that 'it can be confusing for translators and respondents how to interpret especially the labels "Fairly satisfied" and "Not very satisfied". In fact, logically one could argue that after the "Very satisfied" category "Not very satisfied" contains all other possible answers and that therefore it is not clear when to use the category of "Fairly satisfied"'.

Research Question Given the foregoing discussion and the results from the HSIS-studies, we address the following research question: Are the response options of the same item in different languages interpreted differently?

Difference in Interpretation Between Different Languages

Several items from the HSIS-studies have been assessed by judges from at least two countries. We have two pairs which were assessed by Spanish and American students, two pairs assessed by Dutch and American students and two pairs which were assessed by students from all three countries. The wording in the language of the source questionnaire the item is taken from is of importance for the comparison of the scale interpretation by these students. If a difference in interpretation is found, than one of the explanations for that difference might lie in the translation, by which the meaning of the response options may have been changed unwillingly.

The two items assessed only by Spanish and American students, are a 3-point item on happiness from the Eurobarometer and a 3-point item on life satisfaction from the International Tension Study. The results of the assessments of the response scales of these items are depicted in Fig. 5.3.

The Spanish students assign almost identical intervals to the response options of the happiness items and the response options of the life satisfaction item. The length of the interval which American students assign to the middle option of both items is nearly the same as the length assigned by the Spanish students. In comparison to the

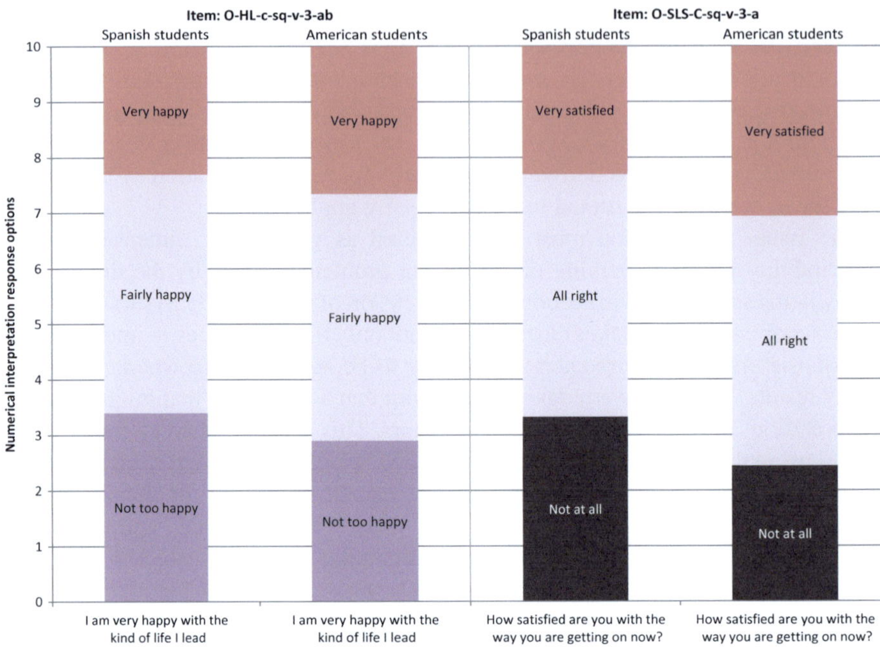

Fig. 5.3 Difference in interpretation between Spanish and American students

Spanish students, the American students reserve a larger part of the continuum for the most positively formulated response options at the cost of the length of the interval assigned to the lower anchor point. This difference between the assessments of the two language groups can have several causes, one of which may be a change in the meaning of the response options after translation into Spanish but then the difference might just as well be indicative for a cultural bias or both.

The two items assessed only by Dutch and American students, are a 5-point Likert item on life satisfaction, but with a leading question on the topic happiness, taken from the European Readers Digest Survey and a 6-point item on happiness which is part of the frequently used health inventory SF-36.[4] The results of the assessments of the response scales of these items are depicted in Fig. 5.4.

Similarly to the results for the Spanish\American student comparison and the discrepancies in interval lengths for positively formulated response options, the American students again reserve a larger part of the continuum for the more positively formulated response options than in this case the Dutch students. The response scale of the item presented on the right side of Fig. 5.4 is an all-inclusive scale. The American students on average assign a smaller length to the interval representing the anchor points than do the Dutch students. This difference could

[4]SF-36 is the abbreviation for the Short Form Health Survey, a set of items developed in the Medical Outcomes Study (Ware and Sherbourne 1992).

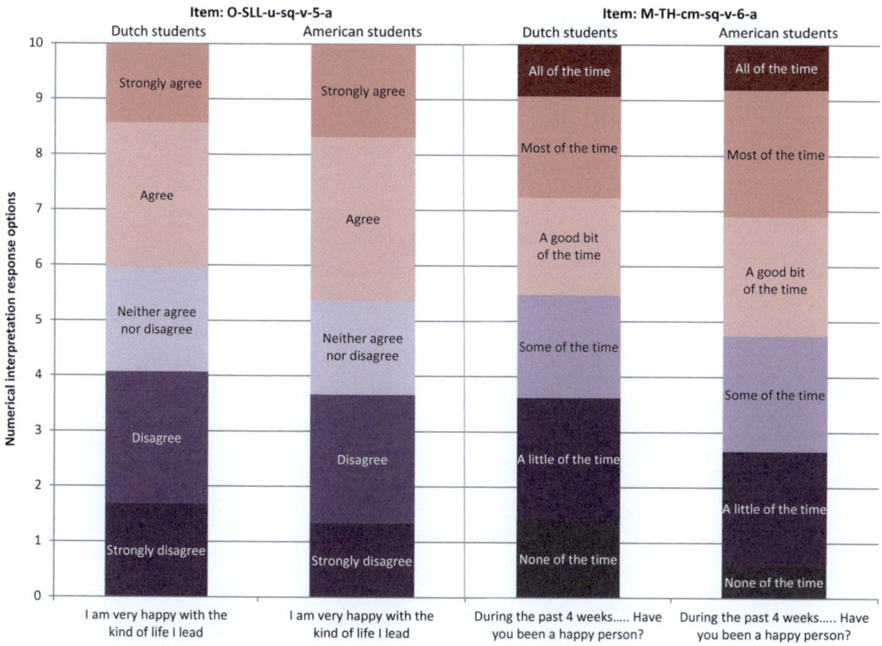

Fig. 5.4 Difference in interpretation between Dutch and American students

point to a difference in culture between the two groups of students, which may cause a larger share of American students than of Dutch students to assign a zero-width interval to the anchor points of an all-inclusive scale. The American students choosing the upper and lower bound equal to one of the extremes of the continuum. Obviously, data on one item is too little to draw general conclusions with respect to this issue. We discuss the assignment of zero-width intervals in more detail in Chap. 6.

The results for the items assessed by all three students groups: Dutch, American and Spanish, are presented in Fig. 5.5. The 4-point item on life satisfaction depicted on the left part of Fig. 5.5 is taken from the Eurobarometer. The 7-point item on happiness which is shown on the right part of Fig. 5.5 is taken from the International Periodical Social Survey Program (ISSP). This 7-point item has an all-inclusive scale, using the adjective ‘Completely’ to label the anchor points.

The results for the Eurobarometer item strengthen the notion that the American students assign a larger part of the continuum for the more positively formulated response options than do the Dutch and the Spanish students. The assessments of the ISSP-scale by the Spanish students do not differ much from the assessments made by the American students. The length of the interval assigned to the anchor points of this all-inclusive scale by students from Spain and the USA is on average clearly smaller than that of the interval assigned by Dutch students.

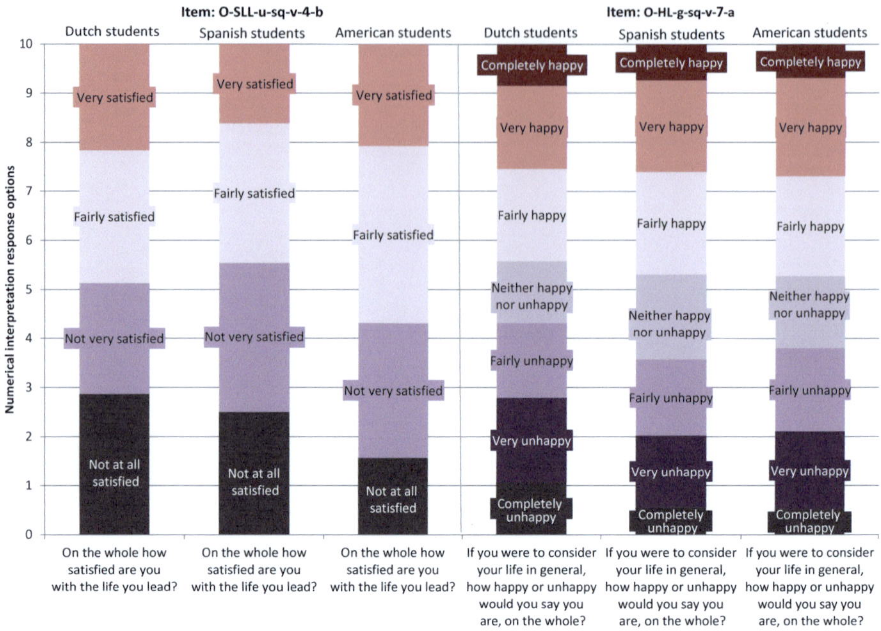

Fig. 5.5 Difference in interpretation between Dutch, Spanish and American students

Different Questions About the Same Topic, But with Identical Response Options

The Leading Question and Comparability

The leading question of a survey item should be formulated in such a way that an answer given by a respondent will be related to the concept that one would like to measure. There are many aspects which have to be taken into account in this respect. Respondents must, among other things, be able to comprehend the question in the way intended by the designer and retrieve from their experiences the relevant information to answer the question (Willis 2004, p. 25). In addition, respondents tend to discard the original words of the question and answer it having placed their own interpretation on the question (Krosnick 1999, p. 547). This leaves the designer of the survey question with a number of choices, they must choose whether to use absolute or comparative statements, how they will stimulate respondents to answer in the question, and have to decide whether to give, or not, extra information in the request (Saris and Gallhofer 2007, p. 31). With this in mind, it is clear that the designing of survey items to be used for measuring certain concepts, is a flexible and evolving process: questions as we first see them change over time, and even within questionnaires, a topic we briefly touched on in section "The incomparability of time series from different surveys and different time periods". For example, there is the variation Gallup introduced in an item to measure life satisfaction with the response options labeled 'Very satisfied', 'Somewhat satisfied', 'Somewhat dissatisfied' and 'Very dissatisfied' and the leading question "In general, how satisfied or dissatisfied are you with the way things are going in your personal life at this time?". Gallup changed the leading question of this item to "Overall, how satisfied are you with your life…?". A variation in the leading question of otherwise identical survey items on the same topic may result in differences in interpretation of the response options by respondents, as discussed in section "Response options labeled in English".

Research Question Given the foregoing and using the results from the HSIS-studies, we address the research question: Are the response options of items which differ in the leading question interpreted differently?

Difference in Interpretation Given a Difference in Leading Question

The HSIS-studies we use cover a total of eight groups of items with identical response scales but with different leading questions, two items from the Dutch HSIS-study and five from the American HSIS-study. The items of the first group from the Dutch study were taken from past surveys of NIPO[5] and were used to measure happiness. The second group of items taken from the Dutch study consists of two Likert items for measuring happiness, the first of which was taken from the European Quality of Life Survey (EQLS). The second item was the same taken from the European Readers Digest Survey which we depicted in Fig. 5.4.[6] The results of the assessments of the response scales of the items from the two Dutch groups are depicted in Fig. 5.6.

The main difference in the leading questions of the items on the left side of Fig. 5.6 is that the leading question of the first item refers to the affective component of happiness using the word 'feel', whereas the second item is formulated from a cognitive perspective through the word 'think'. Looking at the length of the intervals for both items, this difference does not seem to affect the interpretations of the response options by Dutch students. The leading question of the first item of the group on the right side of Fig. 5.6 refers to a state of life. This is a difference compared to the leading question of the second item, which wording refers to the activity of leading one's life. It is likely that this difference is explanatory for the unequal assessments of the response options of both items. Furthermore, in the items of the first pair of Fig. 5.6 direct questions are used, which are very different

[5]NIPO, the Dutch Institute for Public Opinion, joined with Taylor, Nelson, Sofres in 1999, a combination which is presently known as TNS NIPO.

[6]The items of this second pair, do not have equal labeled response options in Dutch, but we consider the wording for both items as equivalent.

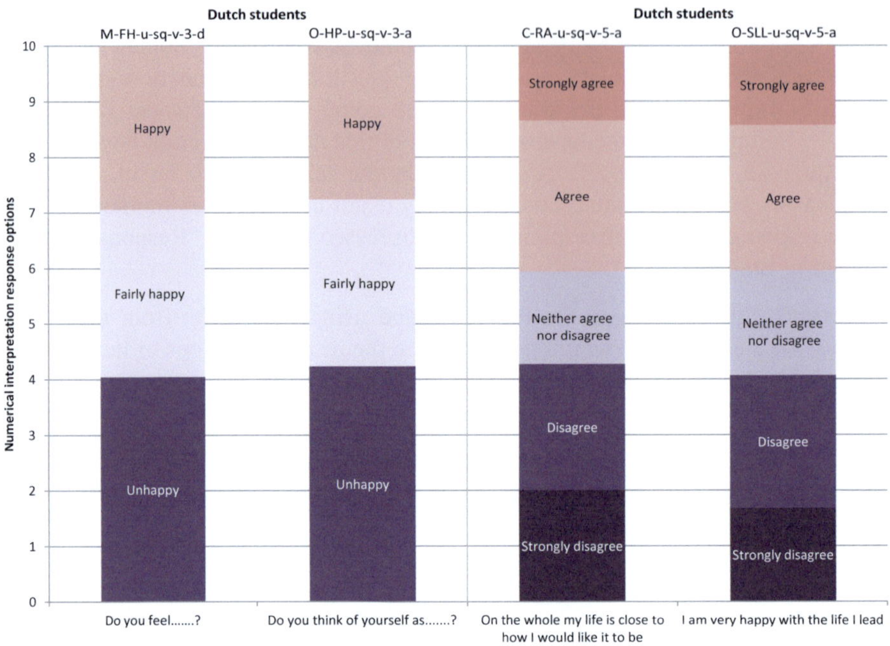

Fig. 5.6 The effect of different leading questions, part 1

from the statements used to pose a question in the second pair of items which have to be answered by ticking Agree/Disagree response options (Saris et al. 2010).

The American HSIS-study covers three pairs of items on happiness which differ in their leading question. The first of these pairs consists of an item taken from the Gallup Poll and an item from the Eurobarometer. An item taken from the Gallup Poll in combination with an item taken from the Canadian General Social Survey makes up the second pair. The third pair with items on happiness is composed of an item taken from the South African Periodical Quality of Life Survey, and part of the fourth pair of items presented in Fig. 4.5, and the item from the Leisure Development Center introduced in Chap. 4. The results for these items on happiness are depicted in Fig. 5.7.

The differences in the leading questions of all of the items shown in Fig. 5.7 do not seem to have affected the interpretation of the response options by respondents. This does, however, not mean that the respondents interpret the leading question of each pair equivalently, but only that if the items are used to measure happiness, the ratings for each item can be mutually compared, without having to correct for a difference in interpretation of the response options.

The two last groups covered in the American HSIS-study refer to life satisfaction. The first group consists of the two items on life satisfaction, part of the item pairs 2 and 3 described in section "Response options labeled in English" and shown in Fig. 4.4. The second group consists of the three items on life satisfaction with

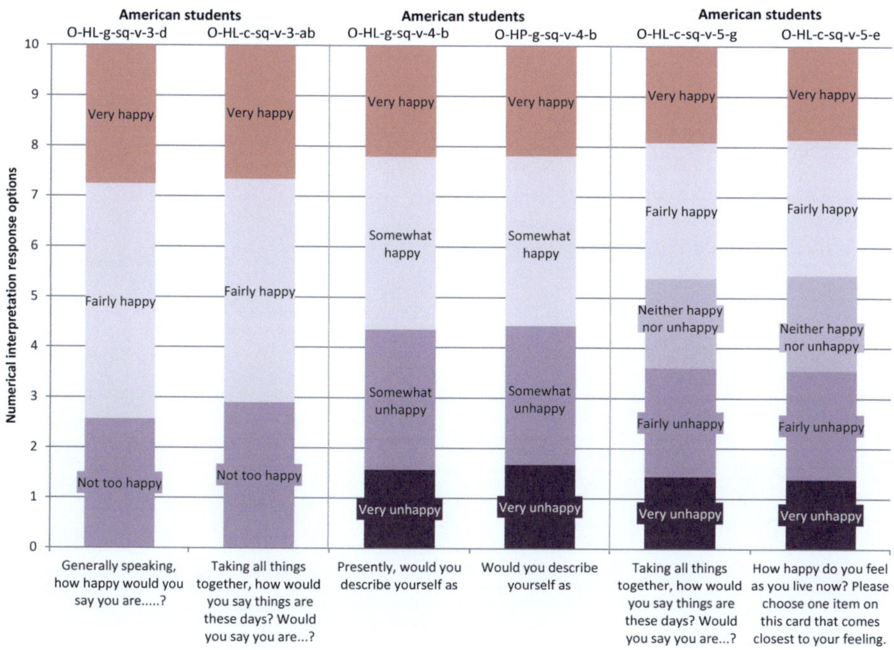

Fig. 5.7 The effect of different leading questions, part 2

5-point scales, shown in Fig. 4.5. The results for these two groups with items on life satisfaction are depicted in Fig. 5.8.

The leading question of the most left item in Fig. 5.8 contains a lot of information for the respondents: the question is about life in general, the contrast between satisfied and dissatisfied, the respondent's personal life and how he or she evaluates this at the present time. Much of this information has been omitted in the wording of the leading question of the second item, which is therefore much shorter. Yet, this does not seem to affect the students' interpretation of the response options. This reasoning also applies to the first two items of the group on the right side of Fig. 5.8. As can been seen from Fig. 5.8, this does not hold for the third item of this group. The response options of this item are interpreted very differently from those of the other two items in the group. This might have to do with the formulation of the question, which, though short, is probably difficult to interpret for respondents. Unlike the questions of the first two items, the question of the third item is less explicit. It is more difficult to know whether the question refers to life in general of to life as a whole, however, we did note that the assessment of this item by the American judges differed from the assessment of the other items by these students. Almost half of the American judges assigned a zero-width interval to the upper anchor point of the scale, by putting the lower bound for this option equal to 10. Moreover, the standard deviation of the assessments by the American students of the upper boundaries of the other response options of this scale, are larger for this

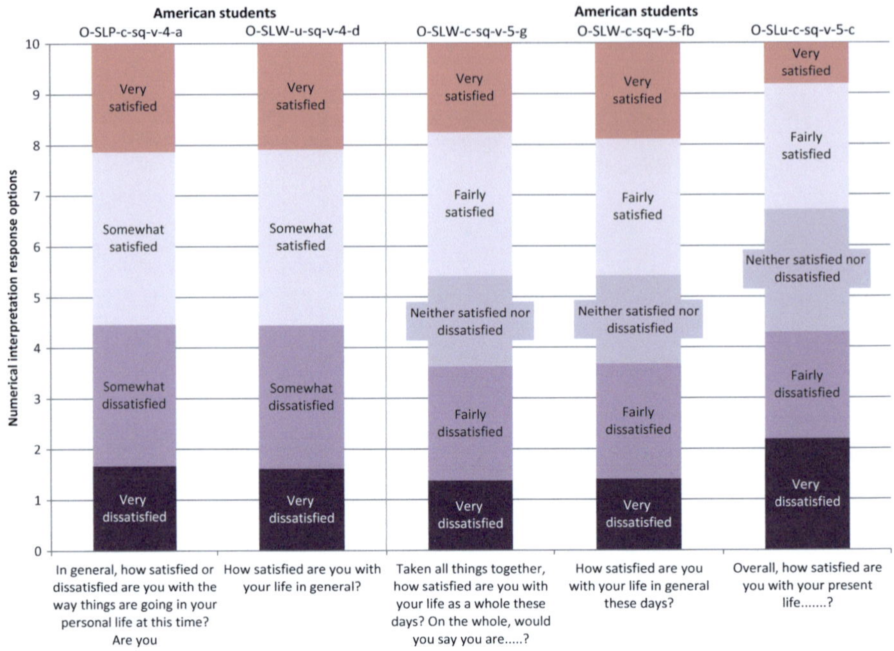

Fig. 5.8 The effect of different leading questions, part 3

third item than for the other two items, as can be seen from Table B.6 of Appendix B. We will discuss the topic of zero-witch intervals in Chap. 6.

Discussion

From the results of the HSIS-studies it is very clear that the meaning assigned to the wording of a response option is to a large extent determined by the context in which the questionnaire is being done, by the language used to ask a question and the working of any response scale.

In most of the examples we had a group of items available all intended to measure the same concept using the same response scales but with different leading questions, we did not find outstanding differences in the students' interpretation of the scale. It is likely that a different formulation which does not change the meaning of a question does not affect how the response options are interpreted.

In the Happiness Scale Interval Study it is assumed that there is no conflict between the personal perception of happiness of a judge and his or her assessment of the response scales (Kalmijn 2010, p. 179). According to Kalmijn, the only justification for retaining this assumption is that it has never been investigated. In addition to this, it is worth noting that, even if the assumption is true, a verbal response scale does not necessarily offer response options that meet the perception of respondents well, such scales may force them to choose between two less than optimal alternatives. The least inappropriate option may be ranked in a counterintuitive position by a respondent who's response falls in between the other response options. As a consequence, the boundaries derived from assessments by judges may not correspond to how response options are selected in practice by respondents. To illustrate this, take the Eurobarometer item with four response options that we presented in Fig. 5.5, which offers the response options 'Fairly satisfied' and 'Very satisfied'. Respondents who are satisfied with their life have to choose between an option that underestimates and an option that overestimates their perception of satisfaction with life.

In this book we do not aim to answer the question of which response scale is the best to use for measure life satisfaction. As early as 1991 Schwarz et al. (1991) made it obvious that the choice of how closed-ended numerical scales are numbered and their anchor points are labeled affects the distribution to survey answers. What we, with the Scale Interval Study contribute, is research that focuses on verbal response scales and provides a systematic way to express the value range denoted by various response options on a continuum from 0 to 10. What our study very clearly reveals is that the degree of happiness denoted by verbal response options, such as 'Happy' or 'Unhappy', is strongly affected by the number of options presented, the wording of these options and sometimes also the position of an option in a response scale. Findings on the same topic obtained using different verbal response scales cannot be compared well.

Conclusion

The degree of happiness denoted by verbal response options, such as 'Happy' or 'Unhappy' is strongly affected by the construction of the response scale used, which is reflected in the number of options presented, the wording of these options and their position on the response scale. The size of the effect may also depend on the language used and the culture of the country in which the item is used. Hence findings on the same topic obtained using different response scales and languages and respondents populations cannot be compared. Conventional methods for scale transformation fail to overcome the differences in degree of happiness or satisfaction with life denoted by the different response options used in different questionnaires. More advanced scale transformation methods or other methods are needed before the findings of individual studies can be used effectively for research synthesis.

References

Braunsberger, B., & Gates, R. (2009). Developing inventories for satisfaction and Likert scales in a service environment. *Journal of Services Marketing, 23*(4), 219–225. doi:10.1108/08876040910965557.

DeJonge, T., Veenhoven, R., & Arends, L. R. (2015). 'Very Happy' is not always equally happy on the meaning of verbal response options in survey questions. *Journal of Happiness Studies, 16* (1), 77–101. DOI: 10.1007-s10902-013-9497-9.

Eurofound. (2010). *5th European working conditions survey: Translation process for the questionnaire.*

Gallup. (2007). *Gallup world poll research design.* Retrieved March 25, 2016, http://media.gallup.com/WorldPoll/PDF/WPResearchDesign091007bleeds.pdf

Harkness, J. A., Villar, A., & Edwards, B. (2010). Translation, adaptation and design. In J. A. Harkness, M. Braun, B. Edwards, T. P. Johnson, L. Lyberg, P. P. Mohler, B. E. Pennell, & T. W. Smith (Eds.), *Survey methods in multinational, multiregional, and multicultural contexts.* Hoboken: Wiley.

Jones, L. V., & Thurstone, L. L. (1955). The psychophysics of semantics. An experimental investigation. *The Journal of Applied Psychology, 39*(1), 31–36.

Kalmijn, W. M. (2010). *Quantification of happiness inequality.* Dissertation, Erasmus University Rotterdam, The Netherlands. Enschede: Ipskamp Drukkers. Available at http://repub.eur.nl/pub/21777

Krosnick, J. A. (1999). Survey research. *Annual Review of Psychology, 50*, 537–567.

McDowell, I. (2006). *Measuring health. A guide to rating scales and questionnaires* (3rd ed.). Oxford: Oxford University Press. http://a4ebm.org/sites/default/files/Measuring%20Health.pdf

Saris, W. E. (1997). Comparability across mode and country. In: W. E. Saris & M. Kaase. (Eds), *Eurobarometer: Measurement instruments for opinions in Europe.* GESIS Nachrichten, ZUMA, Spezial Band 2, Mannheim.

Saris, W. E., & Gallhofer, I. N. (2007). Estimation of the effects of measurement characteristics on the quality of survey questions. *Survey Research Methods, 1*(1), 29–43.

Saris, W. E., Revilla, M., Krosnick, J. A., & Shaeffer, E. M. (2010). Comparing questions with agree/disagree response options to questions with item-specific response options. *Survey Research Methods, 4*(1), 67–69, ISSN 1864-3361.

Schwarz, N., Knauper, B., Hippler, H. J., Noelle-Neumann, E., & Clark, W. (1991). Rating scales: Numeric values may change the meaning of scale labels. *Public Opinion Quarterly, 55*, 570–582. http://www.jstor.org-stable-2749407

Veenhoven, R. (1993). *Happiness in nations, subjective appreciation of life in 56 nations, 1946–1992* (Studies in social-cultural transformation, Vol. 2). Risbo: Erasmus University Rotterdam, Netherlands. Available at: https://personal.eur.nl/veenhoven/Pub1990s/93b-con.html

Ware, J. E., & Sherbourne, C. D. (1992). The MOS 36-item short-form health survey (SF-36): I. Conceptual framework and item selection. *Medical Care, 30*(6), 473–483.

Willis, G. B. (2004). Cognitive interviewing revisited: A useful technique, in theory? In S. Presser, J. M. Rothgeb, M. P. Couper, J. T. Lessler, E. Martin, J. Martin, & E. Singer (Eds.), *Methods for testing and evaluating survey questionnaires* (pp. 23–44). Hoboken: Wiley-Interscience.

Chapter 6
The Labeling of Anchor Points and the Occurrence of Zero-Width Intervals

Anchor Points and Zero-Width Intervals

The labels of the anchor points of a verbal response scale are used to define whether a scale is all-inclusive or not. We consider a response scale to be all-inclusive if there is no wording that is more extreme than the wording used for the anchor points, thus offering room to every possible degree of perception of a given topic. Examples of such extreme wording for the labels of anchor points are 'Completely satisfied', 'Not at all satisfied', 'Extraordinary happy' and 'None of the time'. A response scale can also be one-sided inclusive, which is the case if only one of the anchor points is labeled using extreme wording. Several examples of such scales are given in the previous chapters, for example, the item on life satisfaction from the survey of Statistics Netherlands with the upper anchor labeled by 'Extraordinary satisfied' and the lower anchor labeled by 'Not very satisfied' depicted in Fig. 4.2. The degree of satisfaction expressed by the upper anchor point of this scale cannot be topped by a more extreme degree, whereas the label used for the lower anchor point leaves room for more extreme lower degrees of life satisfaction. An example of a scale which is one-sided inclusive at the lower part is the life satisfaction item from the Eurobarometer, with a non-extreme upper anchor point labeled by 'Very satisfied' and an extreme lower anchor point labeled by 'Not at all satisfied'. This item returns frequently as an exemplar in this book and is depicted in Fig. 5.5. The 7-point response scale of the happiness item taken from the International Periodical Social Survey Program shown in Fig. 5.5 is an example of an all-inclusive scale, in which both anchor points aew labeled using the adverb 'Completely'.

The labels of the anchor points may influence the overall distribution of the responses (OECD 2013, p. 82). Response options formulated with wordings such as 'Completely' or 'Extraordinarily' may tempt judges participating in HSIS-studies to assign a zero-width interval to these options by choosing the upper and lower bound both equal to one of the extremes of the continuum (Kalmijn 2010, p. 147 sqq).

T. de Jonge et al., *Diversity in Survey Questions on the Same Topic*, Social Indicators Research Series 68, DOI 10.1007/978-3-319-53261-5_6

Research Question In this chapter we will address the research question: Is there a relation between the labeling of anchor points and the assignment of zero-width intervals to response options by judges?

The Occurrence of Zero-Width Intervals

For all of the items covered in the HSIS-studies referred to in this book we counted the number of judges who assigned a zero-width interval to the lower anchor point of the scale and the number of judges who assigned a zero-width interval to the upper anchor point of the scale. We have included these numbers in the last column of each of the Tables B.1–B.7 in Appendix B. In addition to this, we also counted how many judges assigned a zero-width interval to both the lower anchor point and the upper anchor point of the scale. We ordered the total percentage of zero-width intervals per item in ascending order for the HSIS-studies conducted in The Netherlands, Spain and the USA and divided the judges into four groups; (1) the percentage of judges who assigned a zero-width interval to the lower anchor point only, (2) the percentage of judges who assigned a zero-width interval to both the lower and the upper anchor point, (3) the percentage of judges who assigned a zero-width interval to the upper anchor point only and (4) the percentage of judges who assigned a zero-width interval to none of the anchor points. The results for these four groups are depicted in Figs. 6.1, 6.2, 6.3, and 6.4. The code given to each item in the WDH is displayed as a reference, as are the labels of the anchor points.

The Dutch HSIS-study covers five all-inclusive response scales. These items, supplemented with the item coded C-RA-u-sq-v-5-c, are also the items with the highest percentages of zero-width items in Fig. 6.1 of which the two scales with more than five response options are at the top. The six items in the top of the ranking differ from the other items in that they have, compared to those other items, a relatively large share of judges who assign a zero-width interval to both anchor points. The appearance of the item coded by C-RA-u-sq.-v-5-c in the top of the ranking in Fig. 6.1 does not seem logical, given that this item at first sight does not seem to have an all-inclusive scale. The relatively high percentage of zero-width intervals assigned to this response scale, may be explained by the fact that for some people, the adverb ‘Strongly’ does not have an added value in this scale which also contains the response options ‘Agree’ and ‘Disagree’. Normally this type of Likert scale is used to ask respondents to state with what intensity they agree with a given statement. For a respondent who agrees with the statement, the option ‘Strongly agree’ might be confusing since it can be interpreted as devaluing the option ‘Agree’ to ‘Not fully agree’.

As can be seen from Fig. 6.1, there are four one-sided inclusive items in the Dutch HSIS-study, two of which have 5-point scales and two of which have 4-point scales. The two items with 5-point scales both use the adverb ‘Extraordinarily’ to label the upper anchor point, and are of particular interest. As we noted in section “An impression of the diversity in survey items”, these scales are rather asymmetric

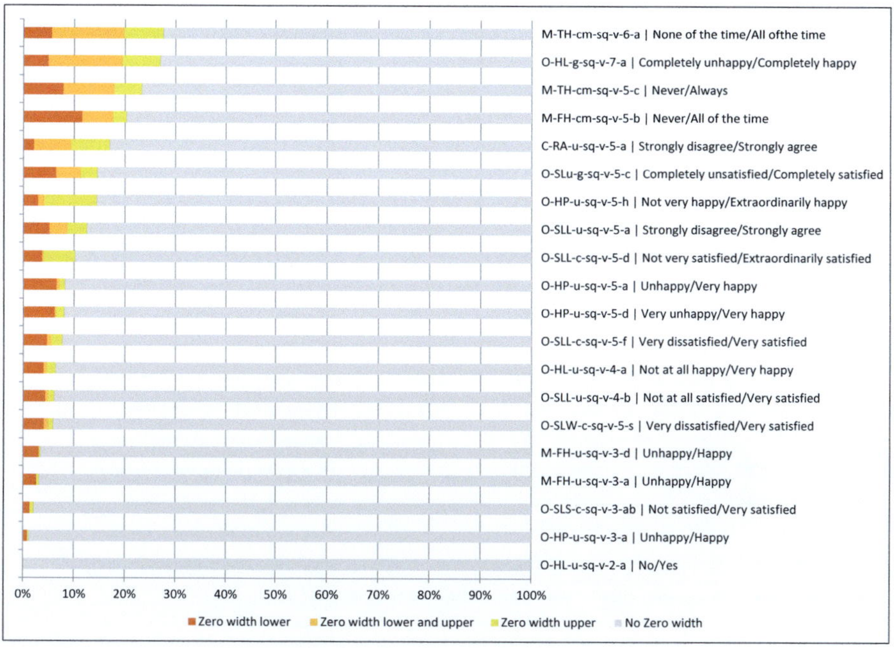

Fig. 6.1 Zero-width intervals assigned by Dutch judges

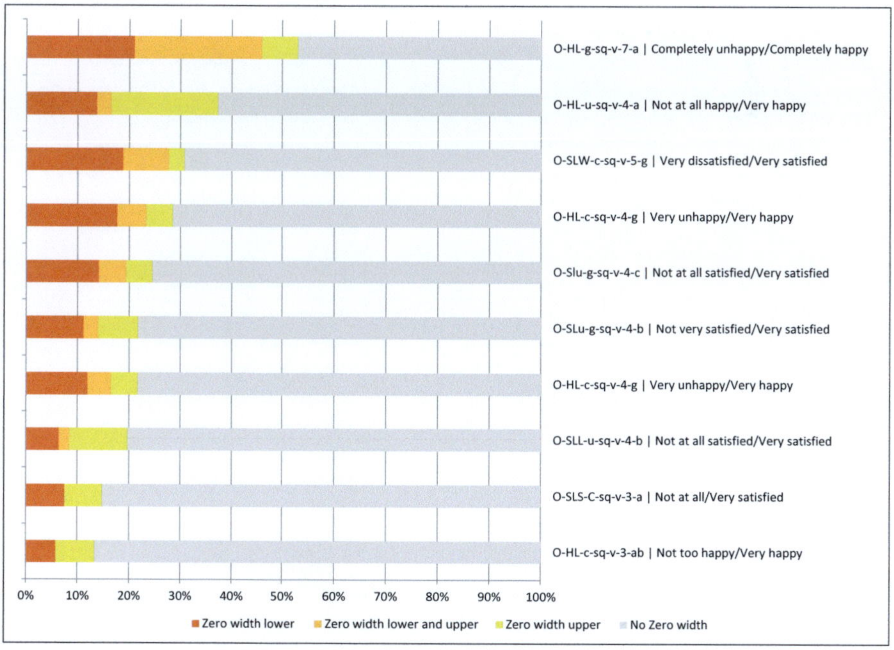

Fig. 6.2 Zero-width intervals assigned by Spanish judges

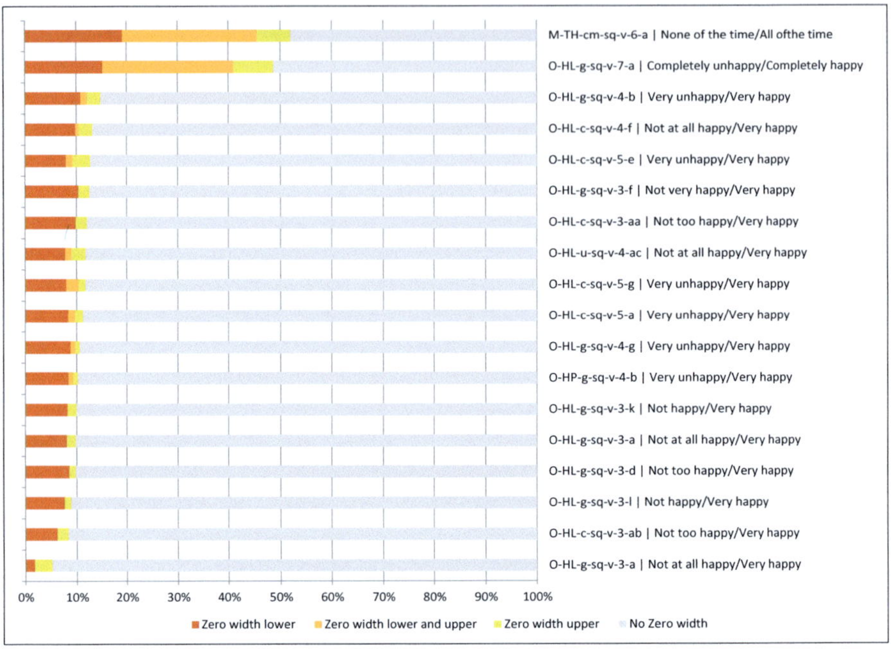

Fig. 6.3 Zero-width intervals assigned by American judges to items on happiness

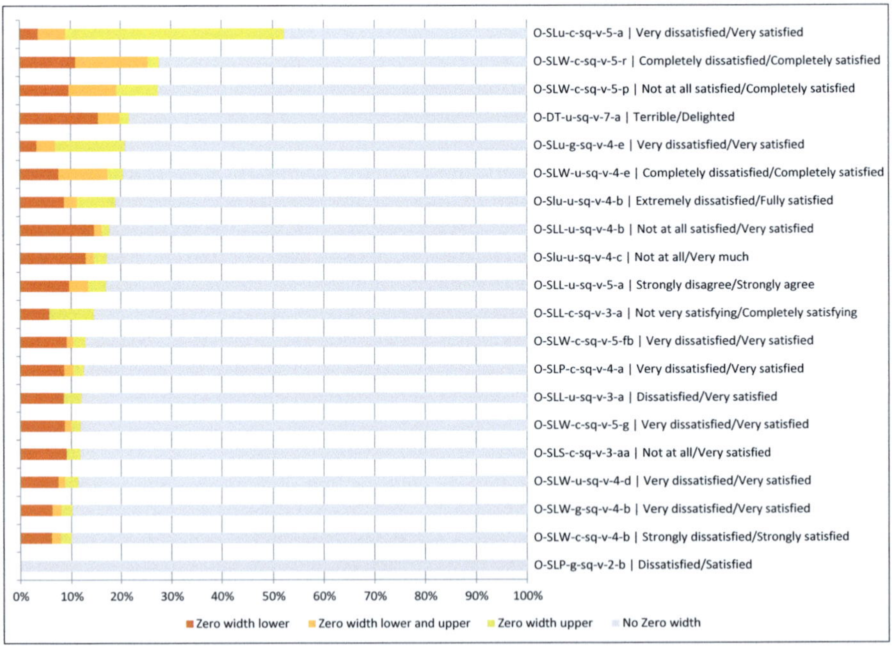

Fig. 6.4 Zero-width intervals assigned by American judges to items on life satisfaction

with only the lower anchor point labeled using negatively formulated wording. Consequently, relatively many of the judges have assigned a zero-width interval to the upper anchor point of these scales, whereas relatively few of the judges have assigned a zero-width interval to the lower anchor point which represents the entire spectrum of degrees of unhappiness/dissatisfaction. It can be seen from Fig. 6.1 that the percentage of zero-width assignments, for the items which have a scale which is neither all-inclusive nor one-sided inclusive, is higher for the lower anchor point than for the upper anchor point. This might be a consequence of the fact that the distribution of happiness and life satisfaction is skewed to the right, which means that respondents mostly rate themselves in the more positive part of the scale and are less used to interpret response options in the lower part of the scale.

Compared to the Dutch and American judges, a larger percentage of Spanish judges on average assigned a zero-width interval to an anchor point of a response scale. The Spanish HSIS-study covers only one all-inclusive item. This is an item with a 7-point response scale, which is, similar to the results for the other studies, ranked on top. Looking at the four one-sided inclusive items covered by the Spanish HSIS-study, the item on happiness comes in at the second place from the top in Fig. 6.2. We repeat the remark made in section "Response options labeled in Spanish" that Spanish people probably rate themselves easier as being satisfied with life than as being happy and consider 'Very happy' to be a more extreme degree of well-being than 'Very satisfied'.

Since the number of items in the American study was too large to present the results for all the items in one figure, we split the results for this study into a set of items on happiness and a set of items on life satisfaction. Two items on happiness from the American HSIS-study were unintentionally doubled and we have left the judgments of these items as obtained in English9 out of Fig. 6.3 but not out of Table B.4 in Appendix B.

The American judges were, in comparison to the Dutch and Spanish judges, relatively moderate in assigning zero-width intervals to anchor points of the response options of the items on happiness, with the exception of the two items with response scales with more than five options. These latter two items were also the only items on happiness with all-inclusive scales covered by the American HSIS-study.

The impression we get from the results for items on life satisfaction included in the American HSIS-study and depicted in Fig. 6.4, differs from that for the items on happiness covered by the same study. We recall from section "The occurrence of zero-width intervals" that almost half of the judges assigned a zero-width interval to the upper anchor point of the response scale of the item on life satisfaction taken from the survey of the Leisure Development Centre (LDC). This result seems spurious, since the scale is not all-inclusive. Looking at the item coded by O-SLu-g-sq-v-4-e, which is on the fifth place from the top in Fig. 6.4, we get a similar impression for a response scale with the same anchor points as the item from the LDC, but one response option less. We do not have an explanation for the large percentage of judges assigning a zero-width interval to both anchor points of these two scales. When ignoring the outcomes for these two items, we find in concurrence with the results in Figs. 6.1, 6.2, and 6.3 that the highest percentages of zero-width intervals in Fig. 6.4 belong to all-inclusive scales, including the Delighted-Terrible scale of Andrews and Withey (1976), pp. 18–19) which we introduced in section "An impression of the diversity in survey items". The percentage of zero-width intervals assigned to the option 'Terrible' of this scale, may be due to the mixture of terms used in this scale to measure a respondent's subjective well-being. This may complicate the interpretation and evaluation of the response options in the context of the scale.

Just as for the Dutch HSIS-study, we notice that the percentage of zero-width intervals is rather high for the Likert item with the extremes 'Strongly disagree' and 'Strongly agree'. It is likely that the high percentage is related to the formulation of the question posed, "I am very happy with the kind of life I lead". Saris and Gallhofer (2007), p. 96) give an explanation which for the Likert item in Fig. 6.4 amounts to the fact that the option 'Strongly agree' is only likely to be chosen by people who have the idea that they are 'Very happy' as prompted by the question and the response options. For people who would be happy to a lower extent than 'very' all other options of this scale could be reasonable choices.

Discussion

A finding which is common to all the HSIS-studies we considered is that the assignment of zero-width intervals to anchor points of response scales occurs more often for the lower anchor points than for the upper anchor points. This might be a consequence of the fact that the distributions of happiness and life satisfaction are skewed to the right, which means that respondents mostly rate themselves in the more positive part of the scale and are less used to interpret response options in the lower part of the scale.

The anchor points of a response scale matter because they set the response frame (OECD 2013, p. 85). They may be helpful to ensure that all respondents understand the anchor points in the same way. It is suggested in the report of the OECD that it would be advisable to use all-inclusive response scales because that would encompass the full spectrum of possible experiences, as this would make it clear where a scale ends. We however, find that all-inclusive response scales encourage judges to assign zero-width intervals to both anchor points, especially when the number of response options is higher than five. In other words, the choice of extremely worded labels for anchor points could make these points more or less redundant. We therefore believe that, in cases where preference is given to a verbal scale over a numerical scale, that either a 5-point scale should be used or that a different, and a less extreme, wording should be chosen for the labeling of the anchor points to give the points enough space on the continuum chosen. When preference is given to a numerical scale over a verbal scale, we consider it more appropriate to label the anchor points in such a manner that they will make the scale all-inclusive by, preferably, using the labels 'Worst possible' and 'Best possible'.

Conclusion

The phenomenon of assigning zero-width intervals occurs more frequently when extreme wording is used for a label of an anchor point and when the response scale consists of more than five response options. Although all-inclusive response scales would encompass the full spectrum of possible experiences, they are likely to make the anchor points on such a scale redundant for part of the respondents.

References

Andrews, F. M., & Withey, S. B. (1976). *Social indicator of well-being, Americans' perceptions of life quality*. New York: Plenum Press.

Kalmijn, W. M. (2010). *Quantification of happiness inequality*. Dissertation, Erasmus University Rotterdam, The Netherlands. Enschede: Ipskamp Drukkers. Available at http://repub.eur.nl/pub/21777

OECD. (2013). *OECD guidelines on measuring subjective well-being*. OECD Publishing. http://dx.doi.org-10.1787-9789264191655-en

Saris, W. E., & Gallhofer, I. N. (2007). *Design, evaluation, and analysis of questionnaires for survey research*. New York: Wiley-Interscience. Wiley Series in Survey Methodology, ISBN 978-0-470-11495-7, e-ISBN 978-0-470-16519-5

Part III
Innovation 2: The Continuum Approach

Chapter 7
The Continuum Approach

Happiness: A Discretely or Continuously Distributed Variable?

We have discussed that neither the two conventional scale transformation methods, Linear Stretch and the Semantic Judgment of Fixed Word Value Method, nor the Scale Interval Method offer a solution to the comparability problem, see Table. 2.2 in section "The three transformation methods and the comparability problem". This has to be attributed to the fact that if a discrete primary scale is transformed by one of these methods, the resulting secondary scale will still be discrete.

Subjective well-being (SWB) is generally understood to be an abstract psychological concept, which cannot be observed directly (Kristoffersen 2015). Latent variables such as happiness and life satisfaction, topics which both fall under the umbrella term of SWB, appear since long and frequently in psychology and social science (Bollen 2002). Bollen discusses a number of statistical models which can be used for latent variable analysis among which are the frequently applied Item Response Theory and Structural Equation Modeling.

In the analysis of survey results, the latent, unobservable variables are normally measured indirectly through observed scores (Kline 2005, p. 60) and it is common practice to use survey items with discrete scales to obtain these observed scores. This use of discrete scales in survey research is often practically motivated, for example in several modes of surveying it is easier to ask a respondent to make a choice from a limited number of options than to have them point out an exact individual value on a continuous scale that corresponds to their perception.

The use of discrete scales in survey research explains the variety of response scales that has been developed over time and, as we have discussed in the foregoing chapters, this variety of response scales limits the comparability of answers to survey questions in general, however, the distribution of unobserved latent variables can be estimated from observed scores, if such scores are obtained using appropriate survey items.

T. de Jonge et al., *Diversity in Survey Questions on the Same Topic*, Social Indicators Research Series 68, DOI 10.1007/978-3-319-53261-5_7

According to Kristoffersen (2015), in SWB research there is a lack of consensus on the metrics of SWB well-being scales. She investigated whether the shape of the response function for life satisfaction might be observed indirectly using the association between life satisfaction and scores measured using the well-known MH5 Mental Health Index which has been constructed such that respondents' observed responses conform to the probabilistic features of the Rasch model. In her paper Kristoffersen gives some illustrations of hypothesized logistic, linear and logit response functions. In this book, however, we will follow a different approach, the Continuum Approach developed by Kalmijn (2010, Ch. VI) to tackle the comparability problem, combining our approach with the notion that happiness has to be treated as a continuous variable.

Outline of the Continuum Approach Applied to Subjective Well-Being

The Continuum Approach postulates a latent SWB variable in the population, which is continuous over the interval [0, 10]. Since the latent SWB variable is unobservable by definition, the same applies to its probability distribution, so one has to postulate at least the type of distribution, which is essentially a decision. In the case of SWB, a beta distribution is the most appropriate choice to use in the Continuum Approach, due to four interesting properties it has (Kalmijn et al. 2011, pp. 509–510)

(i) A beta distribution is a continuous distribution, which makes it suitable as a model for the continuous latent SWB variable in a population
(ii) The random variable of the beta distribution has a two-sided bounded domain, which makes it suitable for happiness as it is measured using two-sided bounded primary scales.
(iii) A beta distribution has two shape parameters, which allows beta distributions to cover a wide class of different distribution shapes, including skew distributions both positive and negative
(iv) A beta distribution is independent of the arbitrary choice of the primary response scale used by the institute that conducts a survey.

We do not know any other distribution with these properties. More generally known alternatives such as the normal distribution and the logistic distribution are less suitable than the beta distribution, among other things because their domains are infinite and they are symmetric around their mean (Kalmijn 2012), whereas SWB has clearly skew distributions (Lee et al. 1982; Cummins 2003; Frijters et al. 2008; Guven et al. 2011).

The family of beta distributions consists of a series of distributions, each member of which is characterized by two shape parameters, α and β.

A beta distribution can be expressed using the complete beta function:

$$B(\alpha,\beta) := \int_0^1 t^{\alpha-1}(1-t)^{\beta-1}dt \tag{7.1}$$

where the parameters α and β are positive real numbers. The symbol ":=" in this context means "is defined as". Given Eq. 7.1 the probability density function of the beta distribution on the continuum from 0 to 10 can be written as:

$$f(x|\alpha,\beta) := \begin{cases} [10B(\alpha,\beta)]^{-1}x^{\alpha-1}(10-x)^{\beta-1} & \text{for } x \in [0,10] \\ 0 & \text{otherwise} \end{cases} \tag{7.2}$$

The mean μ of a beta distribution with parameters α and β on the continuum from 0 to 10 is equal to:

$$\mu = 10\frac{\alpha}{\alpha+\beta} \tag{7.3}$$

To make this less abstract we give some examples of the cumulative distribution functions and the probability density functions for different values of α and β in Fig. 7.1.

If α<β, the probability density function is skewed to the right, if α>β, the function is skewed to the left and if both parameters are equal the function is symmetric about x = 5, the abscissa x being the SWB value on a 0–10 continuum. The larger the values of α and β, the more peaked the density curve and the steeper the cumulative distribution curve.

A starting point for the Continuum Approach to SWB is provided by the cumulative frequencies of measured SWB on a discrete primary scale and the values on the continuum from 0 to 10 at which respondents change their judgment from one to the adjacent response option on this primary scale, for example from 'Happy' to 'Very happy'. On basis of the cumulative frequencies and the values on the continuum of the boundaries between the response options of the primary scale, the shape parameters α and β of the best fit beta distribution are estimated in the Continuum Approach as maximum likelihood estimators. The maximum likelihood estimators of the parameters α and β can be converted easily into the estimated population mean using Eq. 7.3. This estimation procedure is described into more detail in Kalmijn (2010; p. 160 sqq). There is always a perfect fit in the case of a primary scale with three response options. If the number of response options is restricted to only two, then there is no single solution: the number of perfectly fit beta distributions is infinite, and use of the Continuum Approach is therefore invalidated. In the case of at least four response options, then in general there will be no perfectly fit beta distribution and the best fit solution should be taken. Those who are interested in the methodological considerations of the Continuum Approach can find more information about it in Kalmijn (2010, Ch. VI) and Kalmijn et al. (2011).

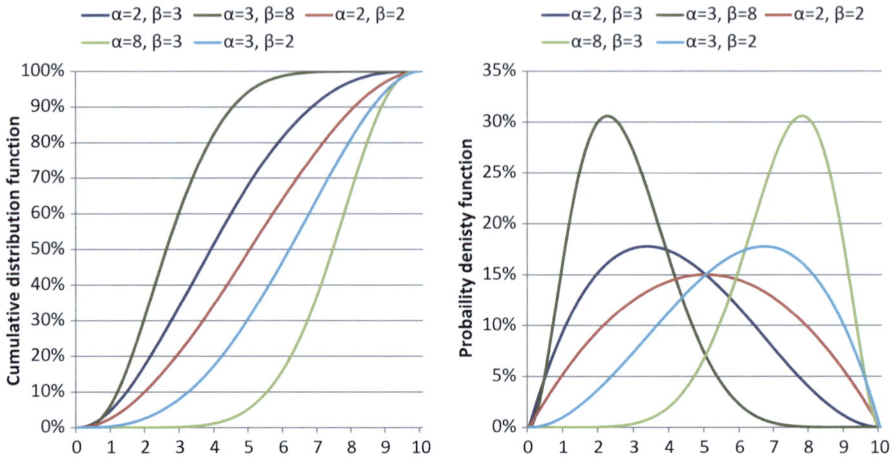

Fig. 7.1 Examples of the cumulative beta distribution functions and the beta probability density functions

Combination of the Continuum Approach with the Scale Interval Method

The two verbal scale items on life satisfaction, one taken from a survey of Statistics Netherlands (CBS) and the other from the Eurobarometer (EB), which we used previously in Table 2.1 to illustrate three transformation methods, are also convenient to demonstrate the application of the Continuum Approach to the upper boundaries of the response options found by using the Scale Interval Method. The average of the upper boundaries assigned by the combination of Dutch students and Dutch employees for these two items and the frequency distribution measured in 2006 are given in Table 7.1.[1] We use the frequency distribution measured in 2006 using these items, to comply with start of the conversion of time series we will describe in Chap. 11.

We used the upper boundaries given in Table 7.1 and the cumulative frequencies based on the frequency distribution for each item in 2006 as input for the application of the Continuum Approach. The result for the CBS item is given in Fig. 7.2 and the result for the EB item in Fig. 7.3. The positions of the vertical lines in both figures on the continuum from 0 to 10 are equal to the upper boundaries given in Table 7.1. The length of each vertical line is equal to the cumulative frequency in 2006 for the response option it belongs to. The continuous line in each figure is the beta distribution that best fits these cumulative frequencies and the given upper boundaries.

[1]The results for the combination of Dutch students and Dutch employees are more representative for the Dutch population, than the results for the Dutch students only. This makes this combination more appropriate to demonstrate the Continuum Approach.

Table 7.1 Average upper boundaries assigned by Dutch students and employees in the Scale Interval Method

Item code survey	Question	Response options	Upper boundaries	Frequencies in 2006
O-SLL-c-sq.-v-5-d CBS	To what extent are you satisfied with the life you currently lead?	Extraordinarily satisfied	10.0	7.8%
		Very satisfied	8.8	33.5%
		Satisfied	7.2	46.3%
		Fairly satisfied	5.3	9.1%
		Not very satisfied	3.6	3.4%
O-SLL-u-sq.-v-4-b EB	On the whole how satisfied are you with the life you lead?	Very satisfied	10.0	47.1%
		Fairly satisfied	7.9	48.0%
		Not very satisfied	5.3	3.8%
		Not at all satisfied	3.0	1.1%

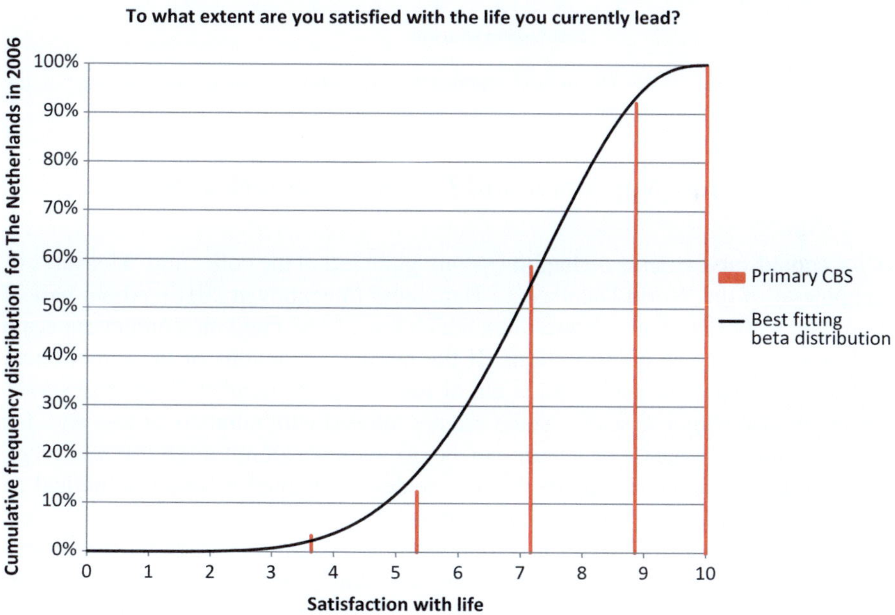

Fig. 7.2 Application of the Continuum Approach to the 2006 frequency distribution for the CBS item

It can be noticed from Figs. 7.2 and 7.3 that the beta distributions estimated for the items of CBS and the EB item do not fit perfectly to the cumulative frequency distribution on the primary scale. We will come back to this in section "Comparison of the estimated means using different methods".

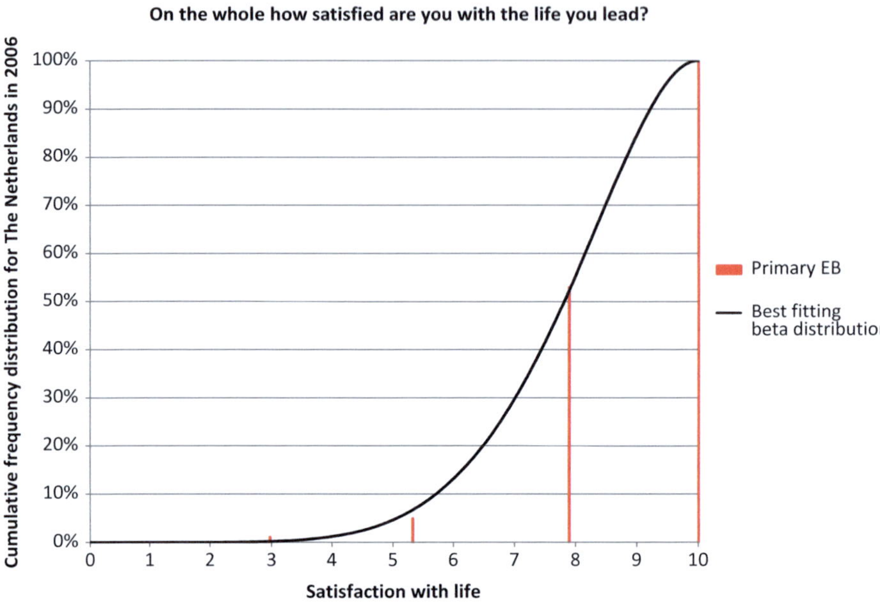

Fig. 7.3 Application of the Continuum Approach to the 2006 frequency distribution for the EB item

The Continuum Approach and Discrete Numerical Scales

All accepted survey items on happiness[2] are gathered in the collection 'Measures of Happiness' of the World Database of Happiness (Veenhoven 2016). About half of these items consist of single questions which have to be rated on a numerical scale with ten or eleven response options. If the number of options of these numerical scales is less than ten, then in three out of four cases the number is equal to seven. There are also response scales which are not labeled with numbers or text and, for example, merely consist of a series of boxes such as □□□□□□□□□□□. When applying the Continuum Approach these scales are treated as quasi numerical as post survey a rank is assigned to each option.

The use of numerical scales is in line with the assumption made by Voorpostel et al. (2009) that attitudes fall along a single, latent continuum and that the larger the number of points on a response scale, the better it represents this underlying, latent continuum and the more accurately it reflects the variation. Voorpostel et al. also state that 'the larger the number of points, the more powerful the scale is in discriminating, but at a certain point respondents become unable to make fine distinctions and thus round off'. In addition, Saris and Gallhofer (2007,

[2]In the WDH the definition of happiness is used in the sense of subjective enjoyment of one's life as a whole, in which definition 'happiness' is synonymous with 'life satisfaction'.

pp. 118–119) mention that respondents who are asked to give an answer on a magnitude scale with fixed reference points, which is comparable to a bounded continuum, have a tendency to prefer numbers which can be divided by five, leading to peaked response distributions. They state that this does not happen if line production scales[3] are used, but that, due to practical considerations when using other modes of surveying, continuous scales may have a future once computer-assisted interviewing becomes more popular.

If the Continuum Approach is to be applied to survey items with numerical scales, a pragmatic choice is to assume that the upper boundaries of the response options on the 0–10 continuum are equidistant (Kalmijn 2013).

We applied the Continuum Approach to frequency distribution measured in The Netherlands in 2006 for the life satisfaction item taken from the World Values Survey (WVS), using the leading question: All things considered, how satisfied are you with your life as-a-whole these days? The answer had to be rated on a 10-point numerical scale from 1 to 10 with the anchor points labeled 'Dissatisfied' and 'Satisfied'. We fixed ten equidistant upper boundaries, one for each response option, starting at 1.0 for the response option at the lower end of the scale and ending at 10.0 for the option at the upper end of the scale as is depicted in Fig. 7.4.

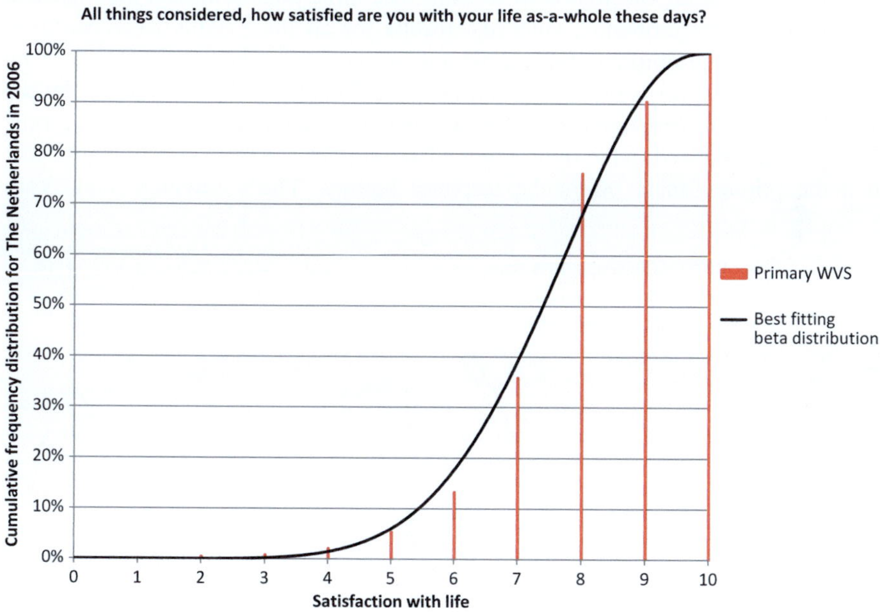

Fig. 7.4 Application of the Continuum Approach to the WVS item

[3]For line production scales respondents are asked to draw a line with a length that expresses the ratio of their judgment to the length of a standard line that is used as a reference judgment for a certain topic.

We have drawn the cumulative frequency measured in 2006 for each response option of the discrete primary WVS scale as a vertical bar at the position of the equidistant boundaries on the horizontal axis of Fig. 7.4. These cumulative frequencies are 0.1%, 0.4%, 0.8%, 2.1%, 5.4%, 13.3%, 35.9%, 76.2%, 90.4% and 100.0%. The curve shown in Fig. 7.4 is the beta distribution that according to the Continuum Approach best fits the boundaries and cumulative frequencies distribution of the WVS item in 2006 for The Netherlands.

The parameters of the beta distribution in Fig. 7.4 are $\alpha = 7.64$ and $\beta = 2.90$, which, using Eq. 7.3, corresponds to an estimated mean of 7.2.

Comparison of the Estimated Means Using Different Methods

We have combined the best fit beta distributions for the items taken from the Dutch versions of the WVS, the CBS and the EB surveys and the frequency distributions measured in 2006 in two graphs which are depicted in Fig. 7.5. The left graph shows the cumulative distribution function, the density function is shown on the right.

As stressed in the discussion in section "The three transformation methods and the comparability problem", since the results for all three items were based on responses made to similar items in 2006, one would expect the three curves to more or less coincide. This is obviously not the case. Comparing the distribution for the WVS item, the distribution for the EB item is too skewed to the left and that for the CBS item too skewed to the right. For the EB item this can be explained by the fact that the primary scale offers the response options 'Fairly satisfied' and 'Very

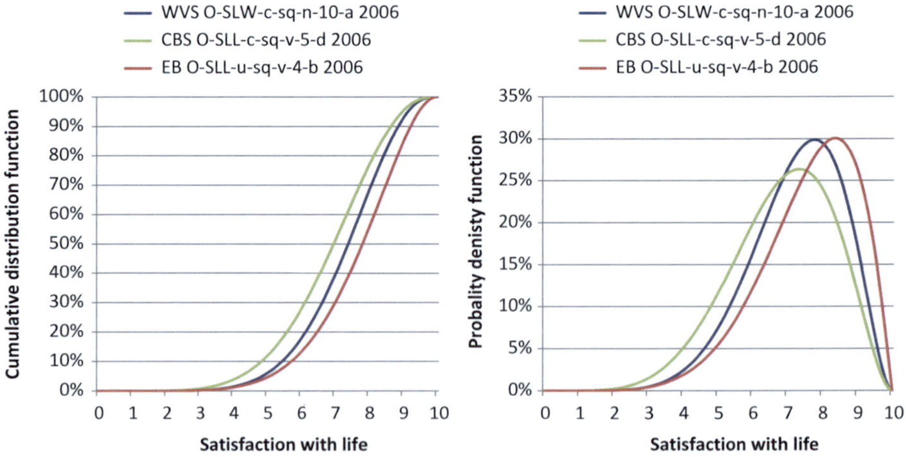

Fig. 7.5 Distribution of life satisfaction in the Netherlands in 2006: estimates using the Scale Interval Method

satisfied'. Respondents who are satisfied with their life thus have to choose between an option that either underestimates or overestimates their perception of satisfaction with life. Apparently a majority of the satisfied respondents tend to prefer the option 'Very satisfied' over the option 'Fairly satisfied', which pushes the beta distribution to the right. The explanation for the CBS item lies in the strong asymmetry of the primary scale in which four of the five options are formulated positively. As a consequence the option 'Satisfied' in the primary verbal scale is positioned in the middle of the scale, which may not be in accordance with the position a satisfied respondent would expect its position to be. Furthermore, as can be seen from Fig. 2.2, the judges valued the position of the option 'Satisfied' in this context rather low on the continuum. As a consequence, the beta distribution for the EB item falls to the left of the distribution for the WVS item.

The estimated population means using the Linear Stretch Method, see section "Linear stretch", the Semantic Judgment of Fixed Word Value Method, see section "Semantic judgment of fixed word value", the Weighted Average Approach, see section "Linear stretch" and the Continuum Approach, see Eq. 7.3, are presented in Table 7.2. The Semantic Judgment of Fixed Word Value Method does not allow the calculation of a mean for the numerical WVS item, since the response options of this item do not contain any words for which the values can be fixed. Based on the discussion on the construction of the primary scale of the CBS item in section "An impression of the diversity in survey items", we can conclude that a mean after scale transformation of 8.5 is far too high to be realistic. We would not expect the mean to be substantially higher than the mean estimated on a basis of the Scale Interval Method for the EB item.

Of all methods that can be used to obtain means, the joined Scale Interval Method and the Weighted Average Approach come closest to the estimated mean for the WVS item. All other methods leave a large gap between the estimated mean and the estimated mean of this WVS item and are far from identical. We can, however, not draw the conclusion from the results given in Table 7.2 that of all methods, the joined Scale Interval Method and the Weighted Average Approach perform best. Previously, in Table 2.2 of section "The three transformation methods and the comparability problem", we presented the means for the EB and the CBS items for the 2008 survey waves, obtained using the first three methods shown in Table 7.2. We found a mean of 6.9 in 2008 for the CBS item and a mean of 7.7 in

Table 7.2 Means in 2006 in The Netherlands according to different estimation methods

Item code survey	Linear stretch	Fixed word value	Scale interval method (weighted average approach)	Scale interval method (continuum approach)
O-SLW-c-sq-n-10-a WVS	7.7	–	7.3	7.3
O-SLL-c-sq-v-5-d CBS	5.8	8.5	7.2	6.8
O-SLL-u-sq-v-4-b EB	8.0	7.7	7.3	7.6

2008 for the EB item using the joined Scale Interval Method and the Weighted Average Approach. This method results in a mean of 7.5 in 2008 for the WVS item. In others words, while the estimated means for the three survey items in 2006 could be considered to be comparable when applying the joined Scale Interval Method and the Weighted Average Approach, this is not the case for the means in 2008. We found similar results for 2008 when the using the item on life satisfaction from the European Social Survey (ESS) for comparison of the item from the WVS (DeJonge et al. 2014, p. 287).

Since the results for the items taken from the Eurobarometer and CBS surveys were the least good compared to other items we looked at, these two items were chosen as illustrative examples to demonstrate that an additional step has to be added to the Scale Interval Method to solve the comparability problem, however, we can conclude that using the Scale Interval Method to transform survey data in general gives a smoother pattern of results than either the Linear Stretch Method or the Semantic Judgment of Fixed Word Value Method. The Scale Interval Method alleviates many of the shortcomings of the two older methods. In contrast to the older methods which do not, the Scale Interval Method does do justice to the continuous nature of the latent variables that are assumed to underlie the survey questions being studied.

References

Bollen, K. A. (2002). Latent variables in psychology and the social sciences. *Annual Review of Psychology, 53*, 605–634.

Cummins, R. A. (2003). Normative life satisfaction: Measurement issues and homeostatic model. *Social Indicators Research, 64*, 225–240.

DeJonge, T., Veenhoven, R., & Arends, L. R. (2014). Homogenizing responses to different survey questions on the same topic. Proposal of a scale homogenization method using a reference distribution. *Social Indicators Research, 117*(1), 275–300. doi:10.1007/s11205-013-0335-6.

Frijters, P., Johnston, D. W., & Shields, M. A. (2008). *Happiness dynamics with quarterly life event data* (IZA Discussion Paper No. 3604).

Guven, C., Senik, C., & Stichnoth, H. (2011). *You can't be happier than your wife. Happiness gaps and divorce* (Paris School of Economics, Working Paper No. 2011–01, halshs-00555427).

Kalmijn, W. M. (2010). *Quantification of happiness inequality*. Dissertation, Erasmus University Rotterdam, The Netherlands. Enschede: Ipskamp Drukkers. Available at http://repub.eur.nl/pub/21777

Kalmijn, W. M. (2012). Happiness is not normally distributed. A comment to Delhey and Kohler. *Social Science Research, 41*(1), 199–202. doi:10.1016/j.ssresearch.2011.11.008.

Kalmijn, W. M. (2013). From discrete 1 to 10 towards continuous 0 to 10: The continuum approach to estimating the distribution of happiness in a nation. *Social Indicators Research, 110*(2), 549–557. doi:10.1007/s11205-011-9943-1.

Kalmijn, W. M., Arends, L. R., & Veenhoven, R. (2011). Happiness scale interval study, methodological considerations. *Social Indicators Research, 102*(3), 497–515. doi:10.1007/s11205-010-9688-2.

Kline, R. B. (2005). *Principles and practice of structural equation modeling* (Series methodology in the social sciences, 2nd edn.). New York: The Guilford Press. ISBN I-59385-075-1 – ISBN 1-57230-690-4.

Kristoffersen, I. (2015). The metrics of subjective wellbeing data: An empirical evaluation of the ordinal and cardinal comparability of life satisfaction scores. *Social Indicators Research* published online: 1 December 2015. doi:10.1007/s11205-015-1200-6.

Lee, H., Kim, K. D., & Shin, D. C. (1982). Perceptions of quality of life in an industrializing country: The case of the Republic of Korea. *Social Indicators Research, 10*, 297–317. doi:10.1007/BF00301097.

Saris, W. E., & Gallhofer, I. N. (2007). *Design, evaluation, and analysis of questionnaires for survey research* (Wiley series in survey methodology) New York: Wiley-Interscience. ISBN 978-0-470-11495-7, e-ISBN 978-0-470-16519-5.

Veenhoven, R. (2016). *Happiness in nations*. World database of happiness, Erasmus University Rotterdam. Available at: http://worlddatabaseofhappiness.eur.nl/hap_nat/nat_fp.php?mode=1

Voorpostel, M., Tillmann, R., Lebert, F., Weaver, B., Kuhn, U., Lipps, O., Ryser, V. A., Schmid, F., & Wernli, B. (2009). *Swiss household panel user guide (1999–2008)*. Swiss Foundation for Research in Social Sciences. Retrieved January 29, 2016, http://aresoas.unil.ch/DataWeb/SHP_USER_GUIDE_W1_W10.pdf

Part IV
Innovation 3: The Reference Distribution Method

Chapter 8
The Reference Distribution Method

Using a Reference Distribution to Derive Boundaries Between Response Options

The observed differences for all methods in estimated distribution means between items as presented in Table 7.2 of Chap. 7 were a trigger to devise a method in which a reference distribution is used to 'tune' responses to other questions on the same topic across surveys.

The Reference Distribution Method for making data comparable builds heavily on the Scale Interval Method. Basically the two methods are identical except that in the Reference Distribution Method the boundaries between the response options of the primary scale are derived from a reference distribution instead of being derived from assessments by judges by means of the Scale Interval Recorder.

With the Reference Distribution Method an attempt is made to deal with the fact that, for a given year and a given population, one would expect the estimated distribution means for similar questions about happiness asked in different representative surveys to be approximately the same irrespective of the primary response scales used: yet as we have shown in the preceding chapters, this is not the case when using the methods described in those chapters. We have explained in section "Comparison of the estimated means using different methods" that this is a by-product of the fact that the verbal scales used in for example the Eurobarometer and CBS items do not necessarily offer response options that meet the perception of respondents well, which forces them to choose between two less than optimal alternatives. The least inappropriate option may be ranked in a counterintuitive position in between the other response options. As a consequence, boundaries derived from assessments made by native language judges may not correspond to how the response options are selected in practice by respondents.

To find a solution to this problem a different angle of approach is needed. Instead of taking verbal scales that have to be transformed as the point of departure, the beta distribution that best fits the survey results of a deliberately chosen item in a given

T. de Jonge et al., *Diversity in Survey Questions on the Same Topic*, Social Indicators Research Series 68, DOI 10.1007/978-3-319-53261-5_8

year is used as the reference distribution to start the transformation of other scales. Preferably, this reference distribution will be based on survey results measured on a continuum from 0 to 10. In general survey results measured on a continuous scale will not be available. As a second best solution a representative survey item with a numerical scale should be selected and used to estimate the best fit beta distribution to can serve as the reference distribution. If the Continuum Approach is used to derive a reference distribution based on survey results measured on a discrete scale, this scale should preferably be numerical with 10–11 response options for the reasons we discussed in section "The continuum approach and discrete numerical scales". If however, only verbal scales are available for types of items that consist of a similar question but vary in scale, one of these items has to be selected as a basis for the reference beta distribution. The Scale Interval Recorder can be deployed to obtain the values of the boundaries between the response options for the selected item. Combined with the frequency distribution for the selected item in a reference year the parameters of the best fit beta distribution can then be estimated and used as the reference distribution.

Once a reference distribution is available, its cumulative distribution function can be used to derive the boundaries between the response options on a continuum from 0 to 10 for any other survey item addressing a similar question, but with a different scale, fielded in the same year as the reference distribution. These boundaries follow straightforwardly from the cumulative distribution of the reference distribution and the cumulative frequencies for the response options in the primary scale: the boundary between response option *i* and response option *i+1* is equal to the point on a continuum from 0 to 10 where the value of the cumulative distribution of the reference distribution is equal to the sum of the frequencies corresponding to the response options 1 up to and including *i* in the primary scale.

The boundaries between the response options are thus determined as the points where the cumulative frequency of the scale in the reference year matches the reference distribution. We refer to the boundaries thus found as reference boundaries, since the reference distribution perfectly fits these boundaries and the cumulative frequency distribution of each other scale in the reference year. The mean of the reference distribution is therefore an estimate of the mean on the 0–10 continuum for each of these other scales in the reference year.

Illustration of Applying the Reference Distribution Method

We described how we applied the Continuum Approach to derive a best fit beta distribution to the 10-point numerical scale and the cumulative frequency distribution in 2006 for the life satisfaction item taken from the World Values Survey (WVS) in section "The continuum approach and discrete numerical scales", and we will now use this best fit beta distribution, which we presented in Fig. 7.4, as a reference for the illustration of the application of the Reference Distribution Method to the life satisfaction item from CBS which we also used in section

"Combination of the continuum approach with the scale interval method". We recall from Table 7.1 that the frequency distribution of the responses to this item in 2006 in The Netherlands is:

Extraordinarily satisfied	7.8%
Very satisfied	33.5%
Satisfied	46.3%
Fairly satisfied	9.1%
Not very satisfied	3.4%

Using the Reference Distribution Method, the procedure to determine the reference boundaries between the response options of the CBS item on the continuum from 0 to 10 is as follows, see also Fig. 8.1.

- We start with the cumulative frequency distribution of the CBS item for which we want to determine where the boundaries between the response options are positioned on the continuum from 0 to 10. This cumulative frequency distribution is shown as a stacked bar on the left side of Fig. 8.1.
- The reference distribution derived from the WVS is depicted to the right side of this stacked bar, plotted against the 0–10 continuum which is represented by the horizontal axis.
- A horizontal line is drawn from the cumulative frequency displayed in the stacked bar on the left side of Fig. 8.1 for each response option of the response scale, to the point where it touches the reference distribution. At this point the value of the reference distribution is equal to the cumulative distribution on the scale of the CBS item.
- A vertical line is drawn latter point to the 0–10 continuum on the horizontal axis. The value at which the vertical line touches the horizontal axis is the position of the reference boundary of the corresponding response option.

Following this procedure, the reference boundaries for the response options of the CBS item on life satisfaction on the 0–10 continuum are, consecutively, 4.6, 5.6, 7.7, 9.0 and 10.0,[1] and, given the reference boundaries at these positions, the reference distribution perfectly fits the cumulative frequency distribution of the CBS item in 2006. The mean 7.2 of the reference distribution derived from the WVS is thus also an estimate of the population mean for 2006 wave of the CBS item.

Reference boundaries found in this way can in their turn be used as input for an application of the Continuum Approach to the cumulative frequencies of the CBS item obtained in other waves. The estimated mean on the 0–10 continuum for each of these waves is equal to the mean of the corresponding best fit beta distribution resulting from the application of the Continuum Approach.

[1]These boundaries are similar to the boundaries we found for the CBS item making use of a reference distribution derivation from item on life satisfaction in the European Social Survey which uses an 11-point numerical scale (DeJonge et al. 2014, p. 295).

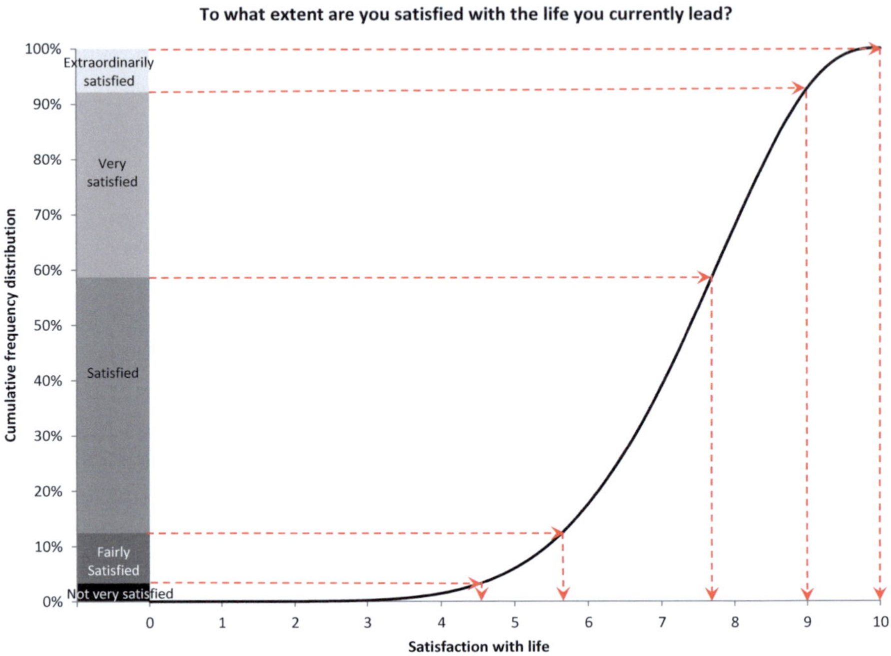

Fig. 8.1 Illustration of the reference distribution method

An obvious question of interest is how the boundaries found using the Reference Distribution Method relate to the boundaries obtained using the Scale Interval Method, where the boundaries are based on assessments made by judges. This relationship is depicted in Fig. 8.2 for the CBS and the EB items which we used as examples in section "Combination of the continuum approach with the scale interval method", to give an impression of what the difference between the two methods means for the positions of the boundaries on the reconfigured scales.

From Fig. 8.2 it can be seen that according to the Scale Interval Method the interval for the response option 'Not very satisfied' in the CBS item, does not overlap with the interval for this option as assessed for the similar option in the EB-item. The latter interval is fully covered by the interval for the response option 'Fairly satisfied' in the CBS item according to the Scale Interval Method. When the boundaries are derived from a reference distribution as done in the Reference Distribution Method, they show a considerable change compared to those obtained using the Scale Interval Method for the CBS item. The boundaries based on the Reference Distribution Method for the CBS scale are more in harmony with those for the EB scale compared to the results obtained using the Scale Interval Method. Using the Reference Distribution Method, the interval for the response option 'Very satisfied' of the EB scale almost coincides with the combination of the intervals for the response options 'Very satisfied' and 'Extraordinarily satisfied'. At the other end of both scales a similar correlation can be noticed for the interval for the

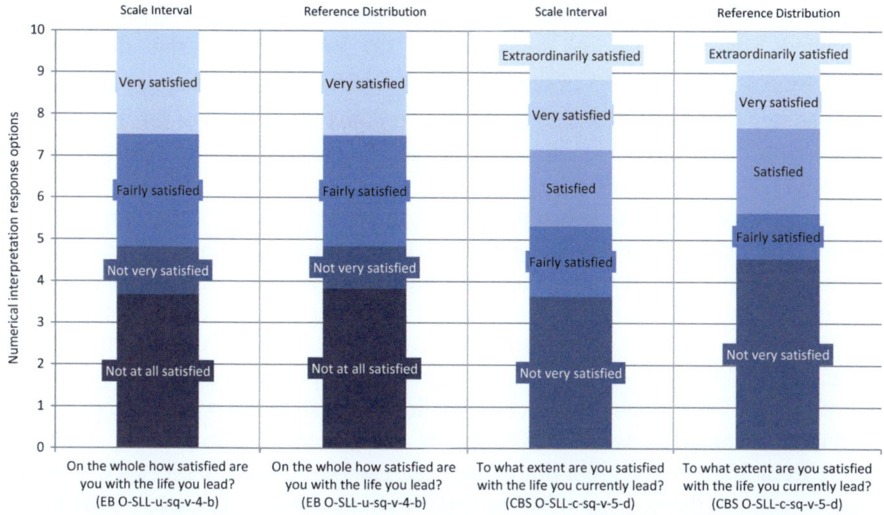

Fig. 8.2 Boundaries as based on the assessments by judges or based on a reference distribution

response option 'Not very satisfied' of the CBS scale with the combined intervals for the response options 'Not at all satisfied' and 'Not very satisfied' of the EB scale.

Scale Transformation Using the Reference Distribution Method

In the Reference Distribution Method the reference distribution used is the beta distribution that best fits best the frequency distribution in a certain year, the reference year, of a happiness item from a deliberately selected survey. Suppose we want to transform the results of another survey for a specific item with a verbal response scale to the continuum from 0 to 10 using the Reference Distribution Method. To do so, given that the results of this other survey have also been measured in the reference year, the positions on the continuum from 0 to 10 of the boundaries between the response options of the specific item can be derived from the reference distribution in the way we illustrated in Fig. 8.1. Once these boundaries have been derived, they are kept fixed in the Reference Distribution Method for the transformation of the survey results for the specific item measured in other years. In other words, to transform survey results for other years, the boundaries remain equal to those derived from the reference distribution for the reference year.

The transformation for each of the other years in which the survey has been fielded consists of estimating the parameters of the best fit beta distribution based on the boundaries derived from the reference distribution and on the frequency distribution of the response on the primary verbal scale in the year in progress. The estimated survey mean is subsequently the outcome of the division of $10{*}\widehat{\alpha}$ by $\widehat{\alpha}+\widehat{\beta}$, see Eq. 7.3 in section "Outline of the continuum approach applied to subjective well-being", with $\widehat{\alpha}$ and $\widehat{\beta}$ the estimated parameters of this best fit beta distribution. The survey results of a whole time series can be transformed in this way.

The mode of surveying, however, does not always remain constant for long lasting time series, it may be changed. If so, it is plausible that this changes or these changes will influence the position of the boundaries between response options. An example of the effect a change in the mode to conduct a survey can have is the Life Situation Survey of SCP in the Netherlands, which in 2004 was changed from face-to-face interviews responding to a questioner to a paper-and-pencil survey using a questionnaire. This mode change caused a dramatic fall in the percentage of people who rated themselves as either 'Happy' or 'Very happy', a drop of 6 percentage points from 2002 to 2004 in a time series that had been rather stable since 1997. In such a situation, the position of the boundaries between the response options has to be reconsidered and presumably determined anew. To derive new boundaries that comply with the new survey mode, the original reference distribution should not be used. Instead the best fit beta distribution given the boundaries derived from the original reference distribution and the frequency distribution of the survey results in the year prior or equal to that in which the mode was changed should be selected as a new reference distribution. Whether the new reference distribution should be based on the survey results for the year the mode was changed or for the year prior to the change, depends on whether there have been two surveys in the year of the change in mode: in the ideal situation a survey will be fielded in both modes to get insight into the effect of the change. In this case the new reference distribution can be based on the survey results for the same year the mode was changed. If unfortunately no double measurements are available, but the survey results show minor changes from year to year, the best fit beta distribution estimated for the year prior to the year the questionnaire mode was changed can be used as a proxy.

In the same way, two different surveys to measure happiness that partially overlap in the years they have been fielded can be transformed and combined if a reference distribution is available for one of them. This reference distribution does not necessarily have to be based on a different (third) survey, but can also be derived from one of the two surveys in question. In this case a reference year has to be selected from the time period in which both surveys were fielded. Next, one of the two surveys should be selected to provide the reference distribution. If the item of interest in this survey has a numerical scale, a reference distribution can be estimated straightforwardly as done for the example taken from the WVS, see section "The continuum approach and discrete numerical scales". If, however, the item has a verbal scale, the boundaries between the response options must be specified first and the Scale Interval Recorder can be used for this purpose. The reference distribution can be estimated using the boundaries obtained using the Scale Interval Recorder and the frequency distribution for the item in the reference year. Once the reference distribution has been found, the time series of both surveys can then be transformed in the same way as we described above.

Application of the Reference Distribution Method

We will now illustrate how the Reference Distribution Method is used by applying it to the items on life satisfaction taken from CBS and EB surveys for results obtained in the Netherlands in the years from 1989 to 2009. This application consists of a trend analysis in terms of the comparability of the trends in responses to different questions about life satisfaction in one country. More elaborate applications of the Reference Distribution Method are given in Chaps. 9, 10, and 11.

In the period 1989–2009, there were two changes in the CBS survey that affected responses. The first change was made in 1994 and consisted primarily of a comprehensive revision of the questionnaire forms and a reduction of the survey items used in several domains. A major change of the survey design of the CBS survey took place in 1997. Primarily, the mode of questioning was changed from paper-and-pencil surveying to face-to-face interviews and, instead of drawing samples based on addresses, the sample for the new protocol was drawn based on individual citizens. This change affected the survey results. In most years of the EB in the period 1989–2009, it was fielded in the spring and autumn, with the exception of 1996 when life satisfaction was not measured in The Netherlands using this survey. To demonstrate the Reference Distribution Method, we averaged the frequency distributions over the EB measurements in a year, to obtain just one EB measurement per year. The means of the CBS and EB items for the period 1989–2009 based on the application of the common Weighted Average Approach are given in Fig. 8.3.

The changes in the design of the CBS survey in 1994 and 1997 are clearly visible in the mean value presented in Fig. 8.3, however, for each of the three periods that can be distinguished for the CBS item, the mean values show a stable pattern.

In most of the years until 1996 the mean value of the EB item was approximately 3.40. In the following years dips were seen in the years 2000 and 2003 and from 2004 the line has climbed to above 3.45 in 2007 and this rise was maintained to 2009.

We used the reference distribution based on the WVS results of 2006 to derive the boundaries between the response options of the items from both the EB and CBS surveys. Using these tuned boundaries we estimated the parameters of the best fit beta distributions for the CBS results over the years 1997–2009 and for the EB results over the years 1989–2009. Fortunately in 1997 the CBS survey was fielded in both the old and the new design, therefore a best fit beta distribution was available based on the survey results for 1997 according to the new design and on the boundaries derived from the WVS reference distribution. We used this best fit beta distribution for 1997 and the survey results over 1997 according to the old design, to derive the boundaries between the response options for the survey results

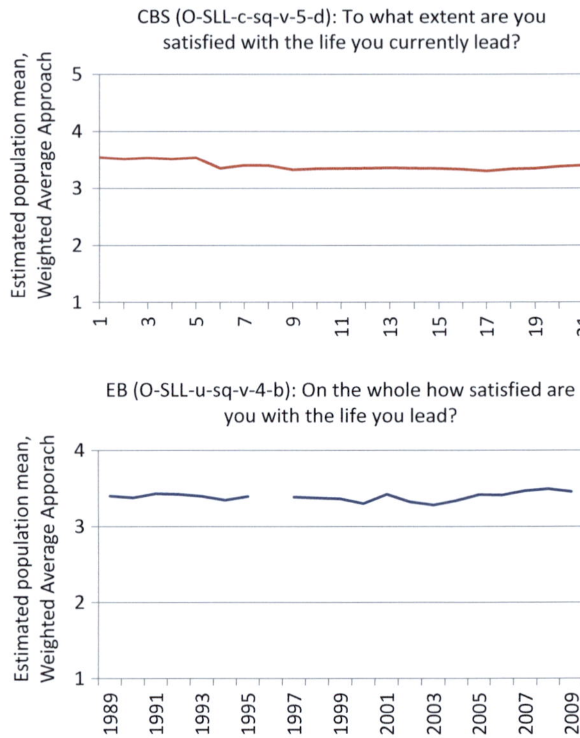

Fig. 8.3 Means of the CBS item and the EB item in 1989–2009 based on ranks primary scale

obtained in the years 1994–1996. In 1993 there was no double survey. Therefore we used the beta distribution estimated for 1993 for the EB as a reference to transform the CBS survey results obtained in the period 1989–1993.

The time-invariant boundaries as assessed by the judges in the Scale Interval Method, the boundaries derived from the reference distribution based on the WVS results for 2006 and the adjusted boundaries for the changes in design for the CBS survey in 1997 and 1993 are given in Table 8.1.

In addition to what is shown for the differences in the position of the boundaries in Fig. 8.2 when comparing the Scale Interval Method and the Reference Distribution Method, we can remark that before the design change of the CBS survey in 1997 the boundaries of the response options in the higher part of the scale were positioned a little lower and those in the lower part of the scale slightly higher. All the boundaries for the period 1989–1993 tuned to the reference distribution for 1993 are positioned somewhat lower on the continuum compared to the boundaries for the period 1994–1996.

The results based on the boundaries obtained from assessments using the Scale Interval Method are shown in Fig. 8.4: for comparison, along with the results for the CBS and the EB items, we have included the results for the WVS item of the survey waves for 1990, 1999, 2006 and 2008.

Table 8.1 Upper boundaries of response options CBS scale and EB scale

		Upper boundaries			
		Judges	Reference distribution		
			WVS	CBS	EB
Item code survey	Response options	HSIS	2006	1997	1993
O-SLL-c-sq-v-5-d CBS	Extraordinarily satisfied	10.0	10.0	10.0	10.0
	Very satisfied	8.8	9.0	8.7	8.6
	Satisfied	7.2	7.7	7.4	7.2
	Fairly satisfied	5.3	5.7	5.7	5.5
	Not very satisfied	3.6	4.6	4.9	4.5
O-SLL-u-sq-v-4-b EB	Very satisfied	10.0	10.0		
	Fairly satisfied	7.9	7.5		
	Not very satisfied	5.3	4.8		
	Not at all satisfied	3.0	3.7		

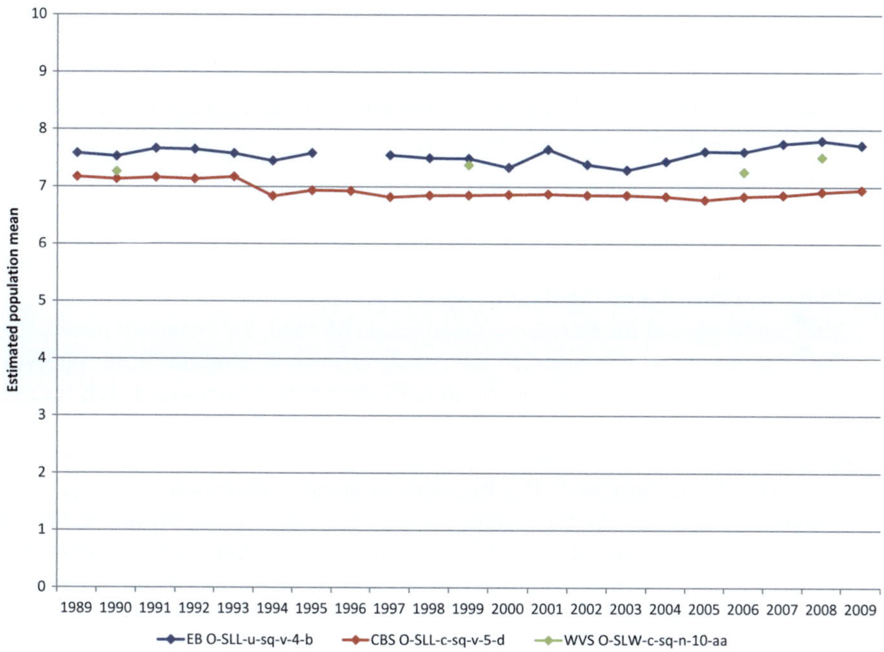

Fig. 8.4 Estimated means using the scale interval method

As can be seen from Fig. 8.4, when the Scale Interval Method is used, compared to the population means estimated for the WVS item, the estimated population means for the EB item are high, whereas they are low for the CBS item. The means for the CBS item when using the Scale Interval Method furthermore show a large discontinuity in the transition from 1993 to 1994 and a small discontinuity in the transition from 1996 to 1997, which are due to changes in the survey design.

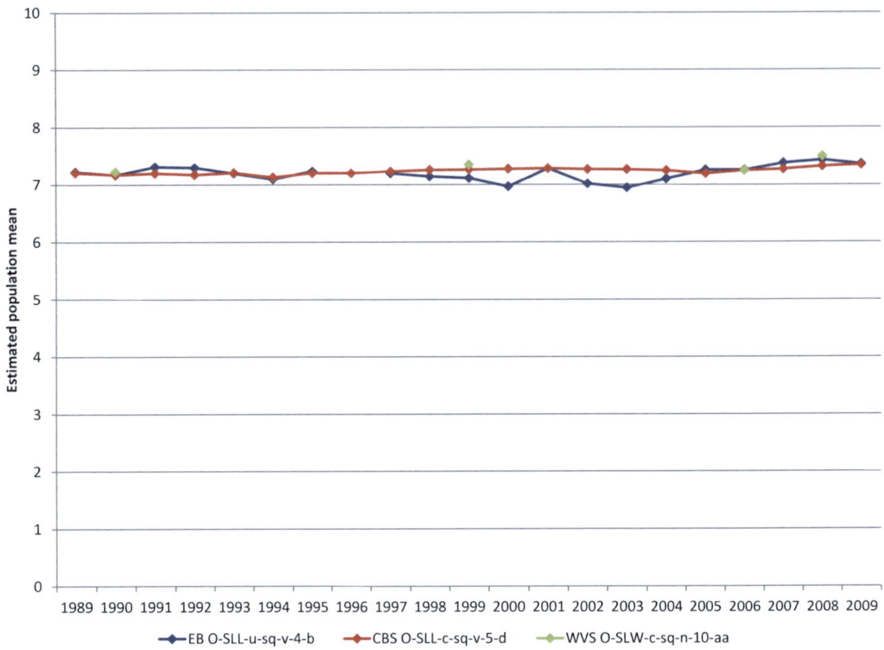

Fig. 8.5 Estimated means using the reference distribution method

We have depicted the estimated means based on boundaries determined using the Reference Distribution Method in Fig. 8.5.

After application of the Reference Distribution Method, the estimated means for the EB item are lower compared to the means estimated using the Scale Interval Method, whereas the Reference Distribution Method causes an upward shift for the CBS results. Due to the adjustment of the boundaries of the response options of the CBS item for 1993 and 1997, the discontinuities from 1993 to 1994 and from 1996 to 1997 have also disappeared. The fluctuations in each survey over the years can now be seen to be similar for the results when the Reference Distribution Method is used and the results obtained using the Scale Interval Method. Application of the Reference Distribution Method results in estimated means for all three surveys which are on a comparable level.

Discussion

In this chapter we introduced the Reference Distribution Method, which in our opinion, provides a valid way to estimate population means based on ratings on verbal and discrete numerical scales at truly comparable levels on a continuum from 0 to 10.

Strengths of Scale Transformation Using a Reference Distribution

The Reference Distribution Method is a variation of the Scale Interval Method and is used to tune survey results to the level of a reference distribution in a reference year. We have shown that this Reference Distribution Method is an effective tool for transforming survey results obtained using different items on the same topic to a comparable scale. In addition, the Reference Distribution Method allows corrections to be made for discontinuities in time series due to changes in the design of a survey. As such the Reference Distribution Method can be used to extend time series as it permits combining results from different surveys that have been fielded in, partly, overlapping periods of time. We discuss this in more detail in Chap. 11.

Limitations

The Reference Distribution Method can be used to correct many of the differences seen in different sets of findings using different survey items on, for example, happiness that are due to differences in the measures used; yet it cannot solve all the comparability problems.

One limitation is that the method requires a reference distribution, typically taken from a same year survey in which the subject to be compared is assessed using a 0–10 numerical scale. If this is not possible, a second best option for transforming distributions on numerical scales is to use the Scale Interval Method, preceded, in the case of a verbal response scale, by a Scale Interval Study.

If a survey has been fielded only once and there is a reference distribution available, then the mean based on the upper boundaries derived from a reference distribution, is by definition, equal to the mean of this reference distribution. This saddles the transformed scores with the errors of the reference distribution, which causes them to become systematic rather than random.

The boundaries between response options that have been derived from a reference distribution are kept fixed as long as the survey design has not undergone a significant change. An obvious question that can be raised is whether it is a reasonable assumption that the boundaries will be more or less stable over time. The answer is affirmative which we will discuss in Chap. 9.

The primary verbal scales of the two items we used in this chapter to illustrate how the Reference Distribution Method works both had more than three response options. The Reference Distribution Method is invalid if a verbal scale has only two response options. There is always a perfectly fit beta distribution, though with zero degrees of freedom, for a primary scale with only three response options. Some 15% of the survey studies on happiness in nations is based on 2- and 3-point response scales (Veenhoven 2011) and thus the Reference Distribution Method cannot be used for making this 15% of survey results comparable with the other 85% of the research findings.

Another limitation is that the Reference Distribution Method is only applicable to the diversity in rating scales, that is, to the last three aspects of the differences in survey questions presented in Table 1.1 of Chap. 1. Survey questions on happiness also differ in the wording of the leading question, such as in the key word used, for example 'happiness' or 'satisfaction with life'. Furthermore, the questions differ also in the time frame that is addressed, some referring to 'current' happiness, while others ask the respondent to appraise 'the last year'. In addition, the Reference Distribution Method has been developed to be applied to single item questions. Yet, there are also multiple question inventories, such as Diener's (Diener et al. 1985) five item 'satisfaction with life scale'. Although each of these items can be tuned in principle, the chance of finding good reference items is lower than that for the case of single items.

Conclusion

Survey studies on the same topic often use different questions. One of these differences is seen in the response scales used, which commonly differ in the number of options available to the respondents in the verbal and numerical scales used and in the words used to label response options or anchor points. As a result much of the available research findings cannot easily be compared. Several methods have been proposed to transform observed scores on these different scales into common scores, typically on a 0–10 numerical scale. All of these methods have limitations and the transformed scores they produce appear to differ substantially from distributions obtained directly using 0–10 numerical scales. The Reference Distribution Method proposed in this book has been shown to perform better than these other methods by bring the estimated population means to a comparable level.

References

DeJonge, T., Veenhoven, R., & Arends, L. R. (2014). Homogenizing responses to different survey questions on the same topic. Proposal of a scale homogenization method using a reference distribution. *Social Indicators Research, 117*(1), 275–300. doi:10.1007/s11205-013-0335-6.

Diener, E., Emmons, R. A., Griffin, S., & Larsen, R. J. (1985). The satisfaction with life scale. *Journal of Personality Assessment, 49*, 71–75.

Veenhoven, R. (2011). *World database of happiness, example of a focused 'Findings Archive'* (RatSWD, Working Paper Series, Working Paper no. 169). Retrieved January 29, 2016, http://www.ratswd.de/download/RatSWD_WP_2011/RatSWD_WP_169.pdf

Chapter 9
Stability of the Boundaries Between Response Options for Different Countries

Research Question

When the Continuum Approach is applied to a time series of a survey which has remained unchanged over time, the transition points are kept fixed. The idea behind this is that, although people may change their perception of the intensity of, for example, their own happiness intensity over time, the assumption can be made that they do not change the value range they attribute to the terms used to label response options. This is an important assumption for research syntheses that require that everything remains unchanged, except for the change of interest. It means that if the Continuum Approach is applied to measurements at distinct points in time, differences in estimates of the mean and standard deviation can be solely attributed to changes in the frequency distributions on the primary scale. Thus the research question addressed in this section is: Is it reasonable to keep the transition points between response options fixed when we apply the Continuum Approach?

We studied this question using two time series on happiness and two time series on life satisfaction based on verbal scale items used in Dutch surveys. The reference distributions for these items came from the items on life satisfaction and happiness found in the European Social Survey (ESS) both with a numerical 11-point scale (DeJonge et al. 2015). Our results were affirmative, but we could only confirm this for the Dutch case. We stressed that further research needs to be done into the stability of the boundaries of survey results obtained in other countries, and that these countries should preferably be countries in which the time has series developed in a different direction from that in The Netherlands. To illustrate this point, we take up the question whether it is reasonable to keep the transition points between response options fixed when we apply the Continuum Approach once more, but now we make use of survey results from two European surveys: the Eurobarometer (EB), which we introduced in section "Three scale transformation methods applied to empirical data", and which is fielded across Europe, and the European Social Survey (ESS). The ESS is an academically driven cross-national

T. de Jonge et al., *Diversity in Survey Questions on the Same Topic*, Social Indicators Research Series 68, DOI 10.1007/978-3-319-53261-5_9

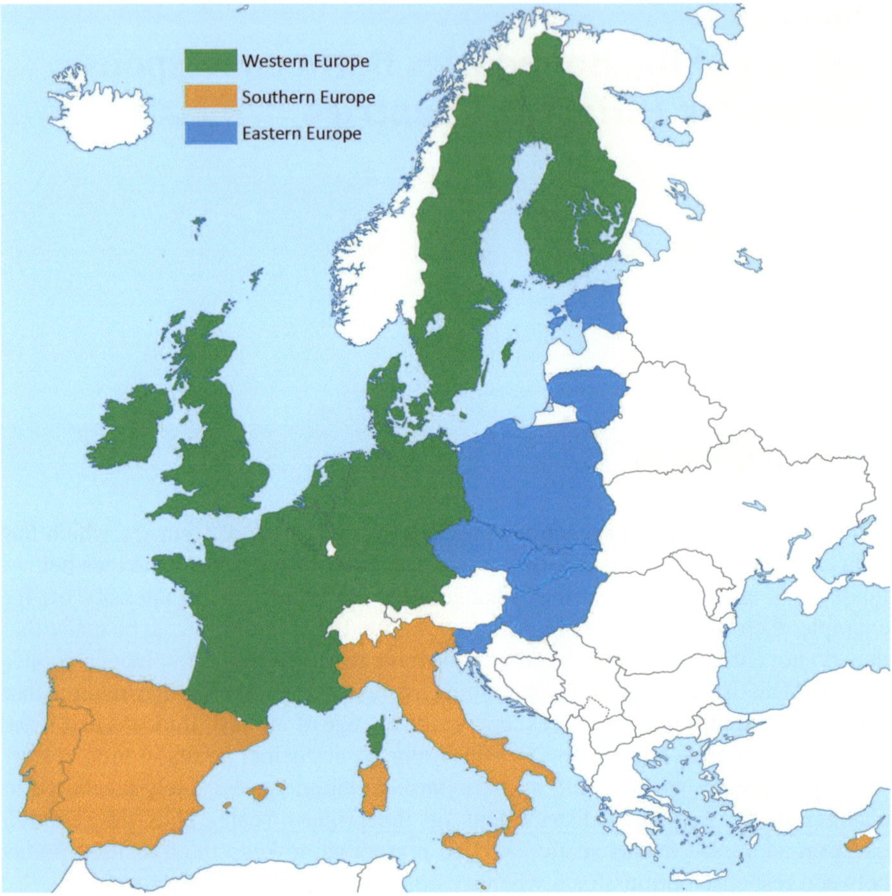

Fig. 9.1 The three groups of countries

survey which was fielded across Europe for the first time in 2002 and since then has been done every 2 years. The ESS is aimed at monitoring social change in Europe. Apart from a question on life satisfaction, both the EB and the ESS also contain a question on satisfaction with the way the democracy works in the country of the particular respondent. We use the latter question to answer the research question, and to address a topic other than life satisfaction or happiness. Both surveys have been fielded in a large number of European countries. For our example we selected all the countries which participated in both surveys in 2012. Three groups of countries could be distinguished, see Fig. 9.1:

Western Europe: Denmark, Sweden, Finland, Germany, Great Britain, Ireland, The Netherlands, Belgium, France, Luxemburg and Austria
Southern Europe: Portugal, Spain, Italy and Cyprus

Eastern Europe: Estonia, Lithuania, Poland, the Czech Republic, Slovakia, Hungary and Slovenia.

We give more details of these surveys in section "Measurements using the ESS and EB items from 2012".

Approach for Testing the Stability of Boundaries

If the Reference Distribution Method is applied, the best fit beta distribution in the reference year by definition coincides with the cumulative frequency distribution of the verbal response scale at the position of the reference boundaries. It is unlikely that this coincidence will also occur exactly for the beta distribution that best fits these reference boundaries and the cumulative frequencies of a verbal scale item measured at different moments in time.

We recall from section "Illustration of applying the reference distribution method" that using the Reference Distribution Method forces the cumulative frequency of a verbal scale item in the reference year into the curve of a corresponding reference distribution and leaves us with a set of reference boundaries. As a result the estimated mean on basis of the verbal scale in the reference year is equal to that of the mean reference distribution.

The main reason for determining the reference boundaries is that they are necessary for the transformation of time series of means based on measurements using verbal scale items into time series of mutually comparable means. To achieve this, the Continuum Approach is applied to estimate the best fit beta distribution for each frequency distribution of a time series of a given item and the reference boundaries for this item derived from the reference distribution in the reference year. In this way we get a series of beta distributions for each item in which every beta distribution is based on the same reference boundaries but each on its own frequency distribution. The reference boundaries are thus kept fixed over time, whereas the frequency distributions vary within each time series. In doing so, we implicitly assume that the boundaries between the response options are stable over time and that the differences in the estimated means can be attributed solely to changes in the frequency distributions on the same verbal scale. When we use the term 'stability of the boundaries between response options over time' we mean that if we apply the Continuum Approach to estimate a beta distribution which best fits the cumulative frequencies positioned at the fixed reference boundaries for a survey item at different moments in time:

- the beta distribution that best fits the frequency distribution of each wave may only slightly deviate from the observed cumulative frequencies at the positions of the reference boundaries
- if there is a deviation, its size should not be related to the length of the period between the time of measurement and the reference year

Examples of the horizontal and vertical deviations of the primary cumulative distribution to the reference distribution at the position of the reference boundaries for two of the response options of an arbitrary verbal response scale are shown in Fig. 9.2.

The horizontal and vertical deviation illustrated in Fig. 9.2 can be formulated formally as follows.

- ***The deviation in horizontal direction:*** for each response option *i* is the difference between reference boundary *i* and the position on the continuum where the cumulative frequency of the response option is equal to the value of the best fit cumulative beta distribution. We will discuss this further in section "Deviation from the reference boundaries in horizontal direction".
- ***The deviation in vertical direction:*** for each response option *i* is the difference between the cumulative frequency of the response option and the value of the best fit cumulative beta distribution at the position of reference boundary *i*. We will discuss this further in section "Deviation from the beta distribution in vertical direction".

If, for a given measurement, both the horizontal deviation and the vertical deviation of the estimated beta distribution to the cumulative frequencies of the primary scale when positioned on the reference boundaries are small, it means that the estimated beta distribution fits well to the measurement on the primary scale. Note: what 'small' means in this context, is a subjective judgment. If, in addition, the standard error of each of the deviations are is small in both directions, than we can confirm the implicit assumption we formulated at the beginning of this section that the boundaries between response options are stable over time and that the differences in transformed means can solely be attributed to changes in the frequency distributions on the primary scale.

Measurements Using the ESS and EB Items from 2012

The item on life satisfaction in the ESS consists of the question "All things considered, how satisfied are you with your life as a whole nowadays" and an 11-point numerical scale with the anchor points labeled by 'Extremely dissatisfied' and 'Extremely dissatisfied'. The item on satisfaction with democracy in the ESS consists of the question "On the whole, how satisfied are you with the way democracy works in your country?" and the same response scale as that used for the item on life satisfaction. To derive a reference distribution for both topics, we only need the frequency distribution for 2012, a year in which both the ESS and the EB were fielded in the countries of our three groups, see section "Research question". The frequency distributions for life satisfaction in 2012 in each group of countries and the corresponding means based on the Weighted Average Approach are presented in Table 9.1.

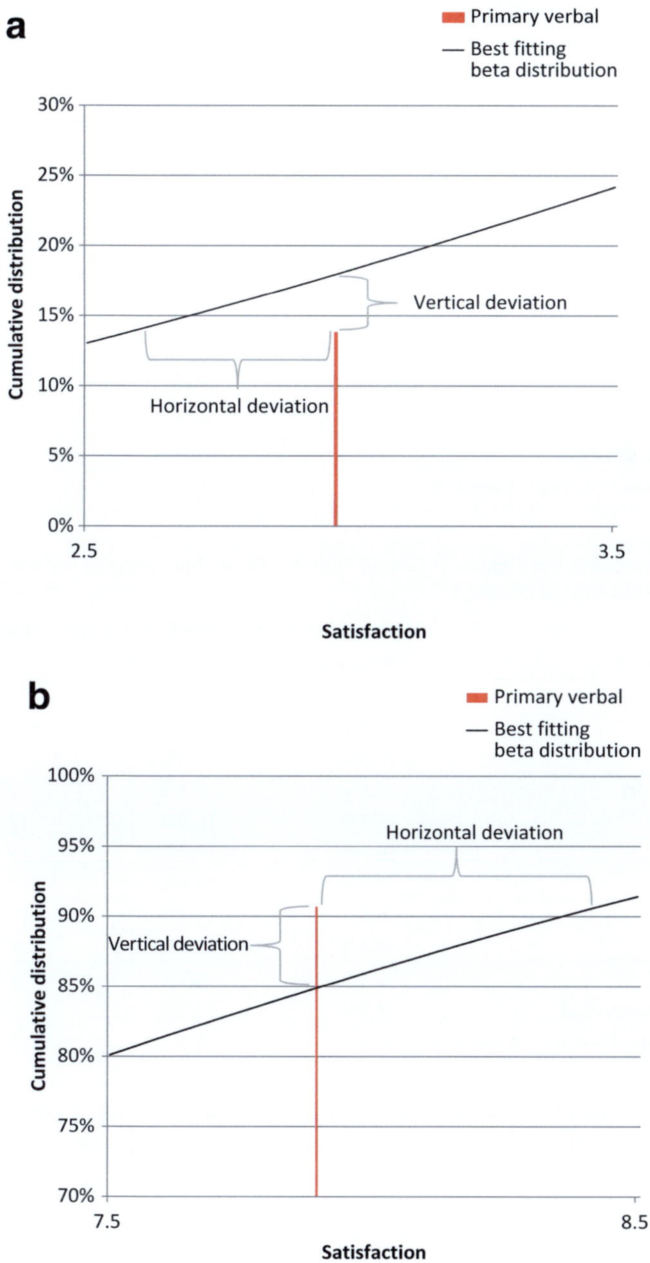

Fig. 9.2 Illustrations **a** and **b** horizontal and vertical deviations

Table 9.1 Frequency distribution 2012 ESS "All things considered, how satisfied are you with your life as a whole nowadays"

Response option	Western Europe (N = 21.952)	Southern Europe (N = 10.031)	Eastern Europe (N = 5.799)
Extremely satisfied	13.0%	11.4%	10.5%
9	17.3%	9.4%	11.7%
8	26.8%	21.5%	21.0%
7	17.1%	18.3%	17.2%
6	7.6%	12.3%	9.5%
5	8.3%	12.4%	13.7%
4	3.2%	4.4%	5.5%
3	3.1%	3.8%	5.4%
2	1.6%	2.5%	2.5%
1	0.7%	0.8%	1.2%
Extremely dissatisfied	1.3%	3.2%	1.8%
Mean, Weighted Average Approach	8.3	7.7	7.7

Table 9.2 Frequency distribution 2012 ESS "On the whole, how satisfied are you with the way democracy works in your country?"

Response option	Western Europe (N = 21.364)	Southern Europe (N = 9.840)	Eastern Europe (N = 5.569)
Extremely satisfied	2.5%	0.8%	1.9%
9	5.9%	1.3%	3.4%
8	16.8%	5.6%	9.1%
7	19.5%	7.8%	12.7%
6	13.8%	10.9%	12.5%
5	16.7%	19.8%	19.0%
4	9.5%	13.6%	12.2%
3	6.6%	13.2%	11.5%
2	4.3%	10.3%	8.1%
1	1.5%	4.7%	4.5%
Extremely dissatisfied	2.9%	12.0%	5.1%
Mean, Weighted Average Approach	6.8	5.0	5.9

Obviously, mean life satisfaction according to the ESS was higher in Western Europe than in Southern Europe or Eastern Europe. Similar information for satisfaction with democracy in 2012 in each group of countries is given in Table 9.2.

As can be seen from Table 9.2, mean satisfaction with democracy in all groups of European countries was lower than mean satisfaction with life. The gap between the means for the two topics is the largest for Southern Europe and equal to 2.7 (7.7 − 5.0), which is to a large extent caused by the high percentage of respondents who are 'Extremely dissatisfied' with the democracy in Southern Europe.

We applied the Continuum Approach to the six frequency distributions given in Tables 9.1 and 9.2 using the method described in section "The continuum approach

Table 9.3 Parameters best fit beta distribution and estimated mean ESS 2012

Group of countries	Topic	Alpha	Beta	Estimated population mean
Western Europe	Life satisfaction	3.22	1.35	7.0
	Satisfaction with democracy	2.73	2.07	5.7
Southern Europe	Life satisfaction	2.35	1.29	6.5
	Satisfaction with democracy	1.52	2.24	4.0
Eastern Europe	Life satisfaction	2.55	1.38	6.5
	Satisfaction with democracy	1.99	2.13	4.8

and discrete numerical scales" for the item of the World Values Survey, to obtain reference distributions for the time series of the EB: we fixed eleven equidistant upper boundaries, one for each response option of the ESS, starting at 0.91 for the response option at the lower end of the scale and ending at 10.0 for the option at the upper end of the scale and estimated a beta distribution that best fits these points for each of the frequency distributions. The parameters of these best fit beta distributions and the estimated population mean for each are given in Table 9.3.

The means in Table 9.3 are lower than those given in Tables 9.1 and 9.2. This is largely caused by the compression of the 11-point response scale of the ESS into the 0-10 continuum.

The EB item on life satisfaction used here is the same item that we used to illustrate the Reference Distribution Method with in Chap. 8. The item on satisfaction with democracy in the EB consists of the question "On the whole how satisfied are you with the way the democracy works in your country?" and the same response options as the item on life satisfaction[1] are used. We used the beta distributions shown in Table 9.3 to derive reference boundaries for the corresponding items from the EB and the frequencies distributions for 2012, these frequency distributions and the reference boundaries for the life satisfaction item are given in Table 9.4.

According to the EB results, mean life satisfaction was, as for the ESS, higher in Western Europe than in the two other parts of Europe in 2012. The frequency distributions and the reference boundaries for satisfaction with democracy item are given in Table 9.5.

The EB results in Table 9.5 show, in line with the observation for the ESS, that satisfaction with democracy in Southern Europe is evidently lower than in Western Europe and Eastern Europe.

[1]Note: the original question in the EB is: On the whole, are you very satisfied, fairly satisfied, not very satisfied or not at all satisfied with the way the democracy works in your country?, but we have shortened this for reasons of readability.

Table 9.4 Frequency distribution EB life satisfaction 2012 and reference boundaries

		On the whole how satisfied are you with the life you lead?			
Group of countries	Topic	Very unsatisfied	Not very satisfied	Fairly satisfied	Very satisfied
Western Europe	Frequency (N = 25.749)	2.0%	7.9%	58.2%	31.9%
	Reference boundary	2.52	4.23	8.28	10.00
Southern Europe	Frequency (N = 6.640)	11.1%	27.5%	53.0%	8.4%
	Reference boundary	3.38	5.96	9.31	10.00
Eastern Europe	Frequency (N = 4.035)	5.9%	20.7%	63.3%	10.1%
	Reference boundary	2.74	5.11	9.14	10.00

Table 9.5 Frequency distribution EB satisfaction with democracy in 2012 and reference boundaries

		On the whole how satisfied are you with the way the democracy works in your country?			
Group of countries	Topic	Very unsatisfied	Not very satisfied	Fairly satisfied	Very satisfied
Western Europe	Frequency (N = 25.378)	8.1%	24.4%	54.1%	13.4%
	Reference boundary	2.60	4.70	8.10	10.00
Southern Europe	Frequency (N = 6.550)	27.7%	43.7%	24.9%	3.7%
	Reference boundary	2.39	5.40	8.25	10.00
Eastern Europe	Frequency (N = 3.954)	17.3%	42.0%	37.1%	3.6%
	Reference boundary	2.51	5.40	8.70	10.00

Frequencies Distributions of the EB Time Series

The EB time series on life satisfaction and satisfaction with democracy for the selected countries span the time period 2004–2015. In this period the EB was fielded almost every year one to three times (European Commission 2012a, b, 2013–2105). An overview of the frequency distributions for the various surveys is given in Fig. 9.3, note: the stack diagrams are projections of the cumulative frequency distributions on the vertical scale.

It can be seen in Fig. 9.3 that the frequencies of the response options in the lower end of the scale, are in each group of countries much higher for satisfaction with democracy than for life satisfaction. The fluctuation pattern over time, by which we mean that the share of respondents that select a certain response option showed considerable variation over the time period of the survey, and this is also stronger for satisfaction with democracy than for satisfaction with life.

We applied the Continuum Approach to estimate a best fit beta distribution for each frequency distribution and the corresponding reference boundaries we derived from the reference distribution for each item. We thus estimated 15 beta

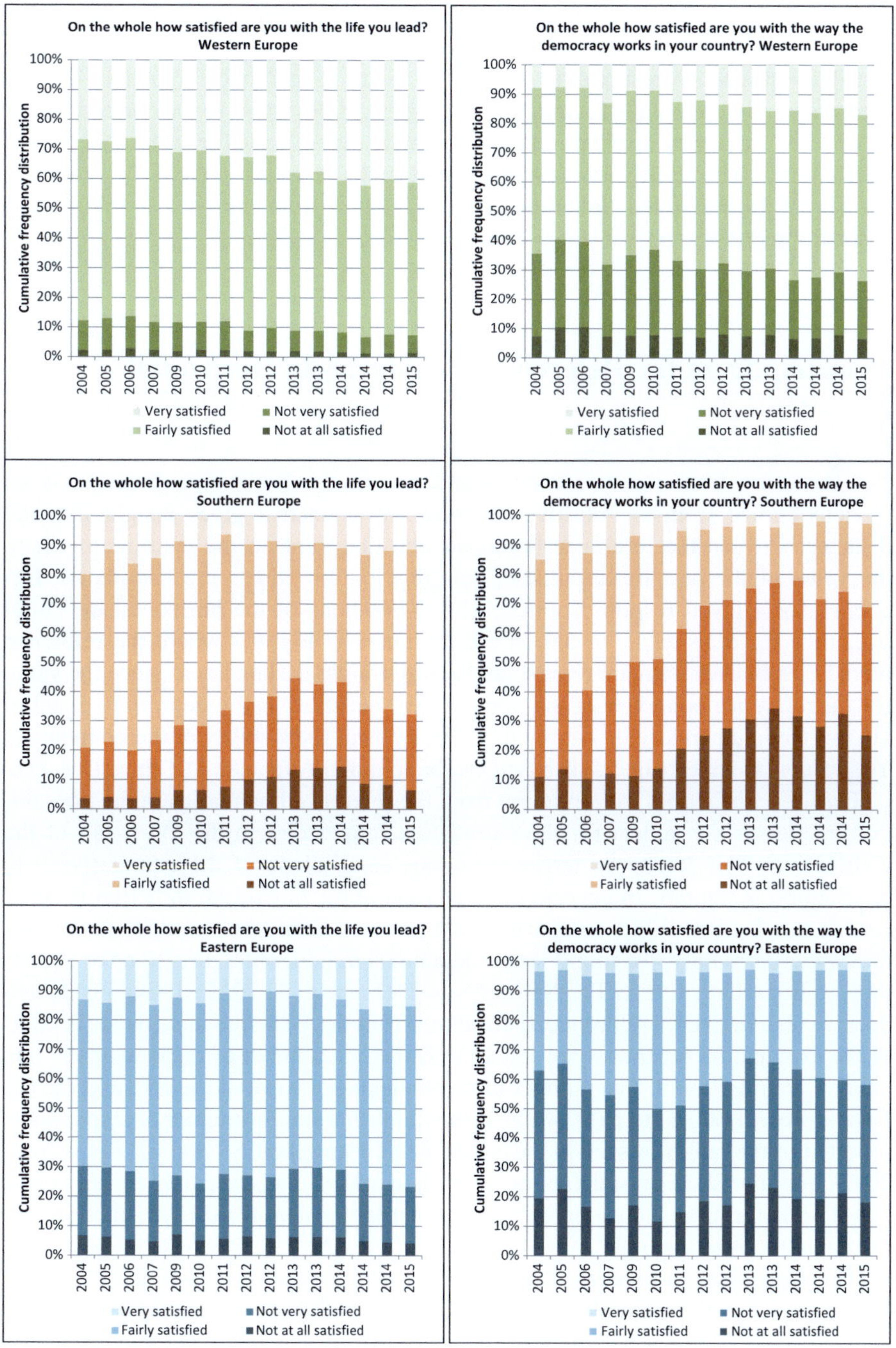

Fig. 9.3 Cumulative frequency distributions EB item 2004–2015

distributions for each item per group of countries. An overview of the cumulative frequencies on the primary scales and of the parameters of the best fit beta distributions and corresponding estimated means is given in Appendix C. We determined the horizontal deviation and the vertical deviation to the corresponding cumulative frequency distribution on the primary verbal scale for each of these beta distributions. The results are described in sections "Deviation from the reference boundaries in horizontal direction" and "Deviation from the beta distribution in vertical direction".

Deviation from the Reference Boundaries in Horizontal Direction

The deviation from the reference boundaries in the horizontal direction is an obvious choice from an intuitive point of view, since it gives insight into the distance between the reference boundary and the point on the continuum where the value of the best fit cumulative beta distribution equals the cumulative frequency for a given response option. The fluctuations of the horizontal deviation over time for each response option are presented in Fig. 9.4 where the reference boundaries of each item are represented using straight dashed lines. Since the value for the reference boundary of the option 'Very satisfied' is, by definition, equal to 10, this trivial boundary is ignored in the analysis of the stability of the boundaries. The values on which Fig. 9.4 is based can be found in Appendix D Tables D.1–D.6.

For life satisfaction, the deviation from the reference boundaries in the horizontal direction is the largest for the cumulative frequencies in the lower tail of the distribution. This has to be attributed to the small slope of the cumulative beta distribution in the tail. In general the deviation in the horizontal direction is small for life satisfaction. When comparing each group of European countries to data for the Netherlands only, we found larger deviations in horizontal direction for the EB item on life satisfaction in The Netherlands (DeJonge et al. 2015). Using just Dutch data we also derived a reference distribution from the ESS data and found that part of the explanation for the larger deviation is that the number of respondents in one country is rather small. The number of respondents per wave of the ESS and the EB is in between 1,000 and 1,500, which is much lower than the number of respondents reported in the tables in section "Measurements using the ESS and EB items from 2012" for the EB. For satisfaction with democracy, the deviation in horizontal direction is for all response options somewhat larger than for life satisfaction, but the deviation is still small.

The frequency distributions of the horizontal deviations from the reference boundaries over the time by year presented in Fig. 9.4, are characterized by their average value, standard deviation and standard error of this average value are presented in Tables 9.6 and 9.7. As a reference we have also included the values of the reference boundaries which we described in section "Measurements using the

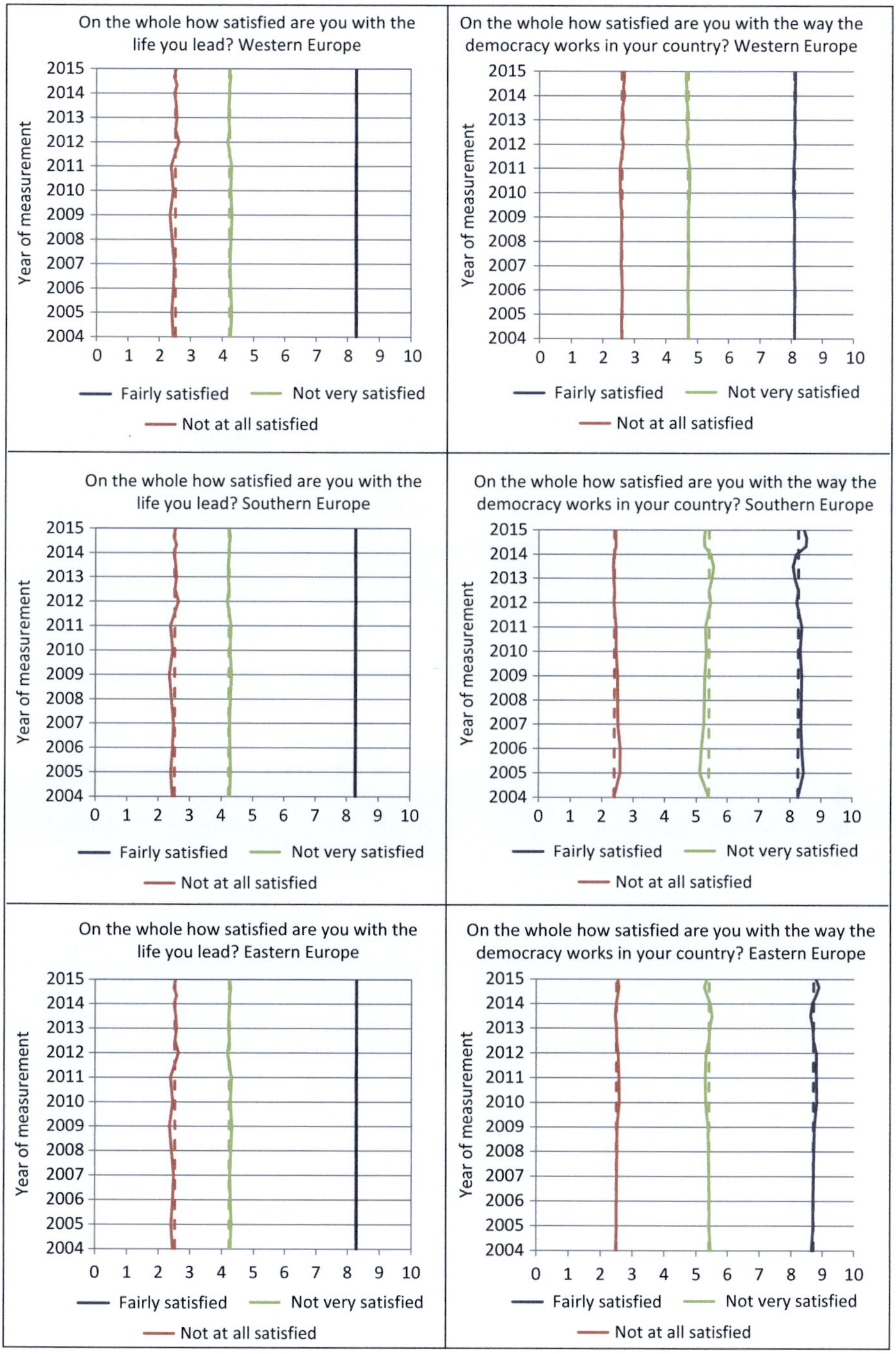

Fig. 9.4 Horizontal deviation to reference boundaries

Table 9.6 Distribution horizontal deviation EB life satisfaction item 2004–2015 (15 waves)

Group of countries	Indicators	On the whole how satisfied are you with the life you lead? Not at all satisfied	Not very satisfied	Fairly satisfied
Western Europe	*Reference boundary*	*2.52*	*4.23*	*8.28*
	Average horizontal deviation	0.032	−0.020	0.002
	Standard deviation	0.08	0.04	0.01
	Standard error	0.02	0.01	<0.01
Southern Europe	*Reference boundary*	*3.38*	*5.96*	*9.31*
	Average horizontal deviation	−0.003	−0.017	0.005
	Standard deviation	0.10	0.09	0.02
	Standard error	0.03	0.02	0.01
Eastern Europe	*Reference boundary*	*2.74*	*5.11*	*9.14*
	Average horizontal deviation	0.127	−0.098	0.024
	Standard deviation	0.07	0.06	0.02
	Standard error	0.02	0.02	<0.01

Table 9.7 Distribution horizontal deviation EB satisfaction with democracy item 2004–2015 (15 waves)

Group of countries	Indicators	On the whole how satisfied are you with the way the democracy works in your country? Not at all satisfied	Not very satisfied	Fairly satisfied
Western Europe	*Reference boundary*	*2.60*	*4.70*	*8.10*
	Average horizontal deviation	−0.017	0.015	−0.005
	Standard deviation	0.04	0.04	0.02
	Standard error	0.01	0.01	<0.01
Southern Europe	*Reference boundary*	*2.39*	*5.40*	*8.25*
	Average horizontal deviation	−0.048	0.075	−0.062
	Standard deviation	0.07	0.13	0.13
	Standard error	0.01	0.02	0.02
Eastern Europe	*Reference boundary*	*2.51*	*5.40*	*8.70*
	Average horizontal deviation	−0.019	0.031	−0.031
	Standard deviation	0.04	0.07	0.07
	Standard error	0.01	0.01	0.01

ESS and EB items from 2012". Below we give an example of how to use the information in these tables: the horizontal deviation of the reference boundary to the cumulative frequency of the response option 'Not at all satisfied' of the item on life satisfaction varies for Western Europe with a standard deviation of 0.08 about an average horizontal deviation of 0.032; this average is estimated with a standard error of 0.02. The horizontal deviation is positive if the value on the 0–10 continuum where the beta distribution is equal to the cumulative frequency is higher than the value of the reference boundary of the corresponding response option.

On average the horizontal deviation from the reference boundaries is small for all the response options of each item. The standard deviation is the largest, with a value of 0.13, for the options 'Not very satisfied' and 'Fairly satisfied' of the item on satisfaction with democracy in Southern Europe.

Deviation from the Beta Distribution in Vertical Direction

The deviation of the beta distribution from the primary frequency distribution at the reference boundaries in vertical direction gives insight into the extent to which the best fit beta distribution under- or overestimates the cumulative frequency of a response option at the position of the corresponding reference boundary. The fluctuations of the vertical deviation over time for each response option are presented in Fig. 9.5. In line with the direction of the deviation, we have, compared to Fig.9.4, interchanged the vertical and horizontal axes to compare the cumulative frequencies of the beta distribution to those measured on the primary verbal scale. Effectively, these latter cumulative frequencies follow the same pattern as in Fig. 9.3, be it that in Fig. 9.5 they are shown as dashed, continuous lines. Since the cumulative frequency for the option 'Very satisfied' is, by definition, equal to 100%, this trivial frequency is ignored in the analysis of the stability of the boundaries. The values on which Fig. 9.5 is based can be found in Appendix D Tables D.1–D.6.

Similar to the deviation in horizontal direction, the vertical deviation from the cumulative frequency on the primary scale for life satisfaction, is the largest for the cumulative frequencies in the lower tail of the distribution but in general small. For satisfaction with democracy, the deviation in vertical direction is, for all response options, larger than that for life satisfaction. This holds especially for Southern Europe. The largest vertical deviation for democracy in Southern Europe is seen for 2005, here it is equal to 4.2 percentage points for the response option 'Fairly satisfied'. This overestimation for the option 'Fairly satisfied', gives an underestimation of 1.8 percentage points for both adjacent options. For the estimated population mean in 2005, this means that the overestimation caused by the vertical deviation for the option 'Fairly satisfied' is, at least in part, compensated by the underestimation caused by the vertical deviation for the other two options. The contribution of each response option to the estimated population mean depends also

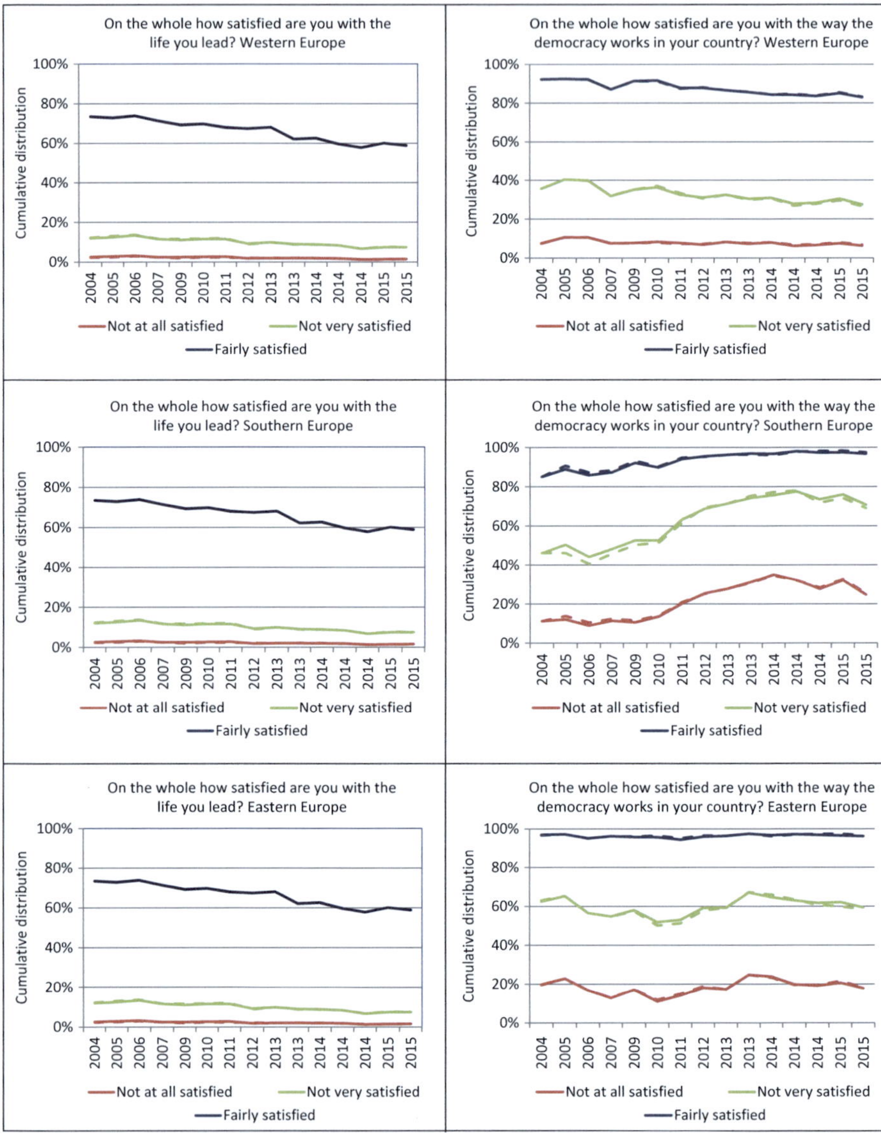

Fig. 9.5 Vertical deviation to cumulative frequencies primary verbal scale

on the distances between the upper boundaries of the response options. This is a topic which we will discuss in more detail in Chap. 10.

We have summarized the vertical deviation of the best fit beta distributions from the cumulative frequencies of each response option of all items by their average, and standard deviation and standard error from this average over the years of the surveys expressed in percentage points in Tables 9.8 and 9.9. Unlike for the

Table 9.8 Distribution vertical deviation EB life satisfaction item 2004–2015 (15 waves)

Group of countries	Indicators	On the whole how satisfied are you with the life you lead? Not at all satisfied	Not very satisfied	Fairly satisfied
Western Europe	Average vertical deviation	0.10%pts	−0.16%pts	0.04%pts
	Standard deviation	0.21%pts	0.27%pts	0.10%pts
	Standard error	0.05%pts	0.07%pts	0.03%pts
Southern Europe	Average vertical deviation	0.07%pts	−0.21%pts	0.06%pts
	Standard deviation	0.56%pts	1.11%pts	0.40%pts
	Standard error	0.15%pts	0.29%pts	0.10%pts
Eastern Europe	Average vertical deviation	0.65%pts	−1.11%pts	0.40%pts
	Standard deviation	0.39%pts	0.68%pts	0.25%pts
	Standard error	0.10%pts	0.18%pts	0.06%pts

Table 9.9 Distribution vertical deviation EB satisfaction with democracy item 2004–2015 (15 waves)

Group of countries	Indicators	On the whole how satisfied are you with the way the democracy works in your country? Not at all satisfied	Not very satisfied	Fairly satisfied
Western Europe	Average vertical deviation	−0.11%pts	0.19%pts	−0.07%pts
	Standard deviation	0.32%pts	0.58%pts	0.22%pts
	Standard error	0.08%pts	0.15%pts	0.06%pts
Southern Europe	Average vertical deviation	−0.47%pts	1.12%pts	−0.48%pts
	Standard deviation	0.69%pts	1.70%pts	0.73%pts
	Standard error	0.18%pts	0.44%pts	0.19%pts
Eastern Europe	Average vertical deviation	−0.21%pts	0.48%pts	−0.19%pts
	Standard deviation	0.44%pts	1.02%pts	0.40%pts
	Standard error	0.11%pts	0.26%pts	0.10%pts

horizontal deviation from the reference boundaries, there is no reference value with which to compare the vertical deviation of the beta distribution from the primary frequency distribution at the reference boundaries. Note: by a positive vertical deviation we refer to an overestimation of the primary cumulative frequency distribution by the beta distribution and by a negative vertical deviation we refer to an underestimation of the primary cumulative frequency distribution.

The average vertical deviation of the reference distribution from the cumulative frequencies is small for all response options of each item, with an also small

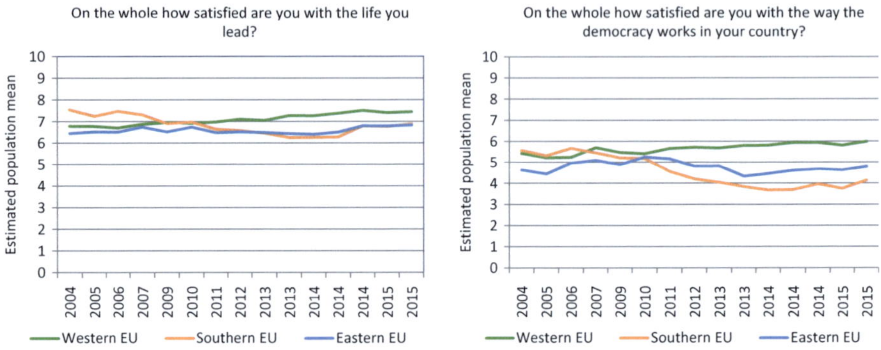

Fig. 9.6 Estimated population means life satisfaction and satisfaction with democracy

standard error. It is worth noting here, that when mutually comparing average vertical deviations for two response options, one should keep in mind that these deviations are related to the cumulative frequencies. For example, the average vertical deviation for the response option 'Fairly satisfied' for the item on life satisfaction in Southern Europe (0.06%pts) is not much smaller than that for the response option 'Not at all satisfied' (0.07%pts), but relatively speaking, the difference between the two average deviations is much larger: the 0.07 percentage points for the option 'Not at all satisfied' which corresponds to an, on average, cumulative frequency of less than 10%, whereas the 0.06 percentage points for the option 'Fairly satisfied' belongs to an, on average, cumulative frequency of almost 90%. Keeping this in mind, the vertical deviations corresponding to the response options on the left side of the scale were relatively larger than those corresponding to the response options on the right side.

In addition to the analysis of the stability of the boundaries, we considered it would be informative to also present the estimated populations means for life satisfaction and satisfaction with democracy by application of the Reference Distribution Method. The means are depicted in Fig. 9.6.

According to what can be seen from Fig. 9.6, life satisfaction and satisfaction with democracy in Western Europe have both increased between 2004 and 2015. In contrast to this, the estimated population means in Southern Europe show a downward trend for both topics, which is strongest for the satisfaction with democracy. Between 2004 and 2015 life satisfaction in Eastern Europe has slightly increased and has come up to the same level as that in Southern Europe. Mean satisfaction with democracy was lowest in Eastern Europe in 2004, but this is positioned between the means for Western Europe and Southern Europe since 2011. In all three groups, satisfaction with democracy lags considerably behind life satisfaction and this has not improved since 2004.

Discussion

The results we found for the horizontal and vertical deviation were similar for both items and groups of countries we considered in this section; for each response option for both items in each group of countries we considered, we found that both the average horizontal deviation and the average vertical of the estimated beta distributions to the cumulative distributions of the primary scales were small. From this we conclude that the beta distributions fit well to the primary distributions. In addition, the standard error of each of the deviations was small. The latter means that the average deviations in both horizontal and vertical direction are stable over time. We conclude that these results confirm the implicit assumption we formulated in section "Approach for testing the stability of boundaries", that the boundaries between response options are stable over time and that the differences in transformed means can solely be attributed to changes in the frequency distributions on the primary scale.

When the Reference Distribution Method is applied, the estimated population mean of the reference distribution serves as a reference value for a comparison of the means of other survey items and other years of measurement estimated using the Continuum Approach. This reference value should not be considered to be the 'true' value of the perception of happiness on the continuum from 0 to 10. If another reference distribution is used, the reference value may be different. In other words, only population means that are estimated using the Continuum Approach to survey items for which the reference boundaries have been derived from the same reference distribution, can be compared.

Conclusion

The question we addressed in this chapter is whether it is reasonable to assume that the positions of the reference boundaries between response options on the continuum from 0 to 10 are stable over time if the Continuum Approach is applied. We conclude that the answer is affirmative, which is in concordance with what we previously found for four different items on life satisfaction and happiness in The Netherlands (DeJonge et al. 2015). In our opinion this justifies the statement that it is valid to use the reference boundaries as fixed values over a longer period of time to make time series on satisfaction based on different surveys comparable.

References

DeJonge, T., Veenhoven, R., Kalmijn, W. M., & Arends, L. R. (2015). Stability of boundaries between response options of response scales. Does 'very happy' remain equally happy over the years? *Social Indicators Research, 123*(1), 241–266. doi:10.1007/s11205-014-0735-2.

European Commission. (2012a). Brussels. European Opinion Research Group (EORG). GESIS Data Archive, Cologne. *Eurobarometer 57.1 (Mar–May 2002)*, ZA3639 Data file Version 1.0.1. doi:10.4232/1.10949; *Eurobarometer 58.1 (Oct–Nov 2002)*, ZA3693 Data file Version 1.0.1. doi:10.4232/1.10953; *Eurobarometer 60.1 (Oct–Nov 2003)*, ZA3938 Data file Version 1.0.1. doi:10.4232/1.10958; *Eurobarometer 62.0 (Oct–Nov 2004)*, ZA4229 Data file Version 1.1.0. doi:10.4232/1.10962.

European Commission (2012b). Brussels. TNS Opinion & Social [Producer]. GESIS Data Archive, Cologne. *Eurobarometer 63.4 (May–Jun 2005)*, ZA4411 Data file Version 1.1.0. doi:10.4232/1.10968; *Eurobarometer 64.2 (Oct–Nov 2005)*, ZA4414 Data file Version 1.1.0. doi:10.4232/1.10970; *Eurobarometer 65.2 (Mar–May 2006)*, ZA4506 Data file Version 1.0.1. doi:10.4232/1.10974; *Eurobarometer 66.1 (Sep–Oct 2006)*, ZA4526 Data file Version 1.0.1. doi:10.4232/1.10980; *Eurobarometer 66.3 (Nov–Dec 2006)*, ZA4528 Data file Version 2.0.1. doi:10.4232/1.10982; *Eurobarometer 67.2 (Apr–May 2007)*, ZA4530 Data file Version 2.1.0. doi:10.4232/1.10984; *Eurobarometer 68.1 (Sep–Nov 2007)*, ZA4565 Data file Version 4.0.1. doi:10.4232/1.10988; *Eurobarometer 70.1 (Oct–Nov 2008)*, ZA4819 Data file Version 3.0.2. doi:10.4232/1.10989; *Eurobarometer 71.2 (May–Jun 2009)*, ZA4972 Data file Version 3.0.2. doi:10.4232/1.10990; *Eurobarometer 72.4 (Oct–Nov 2009)*, ZA4994 Data file Version 3.0.0. doi:10.4232/1.11141; *Eurobarometer 73.4 (May 2010)*, ZA5234 Data file Version 2.0.1. doi:10.4232/1.11479; *Eurobarometer 76.3 (2011)*, ZA5567 Data file Version 1.0.0. doi:10.4232/1.11448.

European Commission (2013–2015). Brussels. TNS Opinion & Social [Producer]. GESIS Data Archive, Cologne. *Eurobarometer 69.2 (Mar–May 2008)*, ZA4744 Data file Version 5.0.0. doi:10.4232/1.11755; *Eurobarometer 71.1 (Jan–Feb 2009)*, ZA4971 Data file Version 4.0.0. doi:10.4232/1.11756; *Eurobarometer 74.2 (2010)*, ZA5449 Data file Version 2.2.0. doi:10.4232/1.11626; *Eurobarometer 75.3 (2011)*, ZA5481 Data file Version 2.0.0. doi:10.4232/1.11768; *Eurobarometer 75.4 (2011)*, ZA5564 Data file Version 3.0.0. doi:10.4232/1.11769; *Eurobarometer 77.3 (2012)*, ZA5612 Data file Version 1.0.0. doi:10.4232/1.11558; *Eurobarometer 77.4 (2012)*, ZA5613 Data file Version 2.0.0. doi:10.4232/1.11697; *Eurobarometer 78.1 (2012)*, ZA5685 Data file Version 1.0.0. doi:10.4232/1.11706; *Eurobarometer 79.3 (2013)*, ZA5689 Data file Version 1.1.0. doi:10.4232/1.12445; *Eurobarometer 80.1 (2013)*, ZA5876 Data file Version 1.0.0. doi:10.4232/1.11881; *Eurobarometer 81.2 (2014)*, ZA5913 Data file Version 1.0.0. doi:10.4232/1.12172; *Eurobarometer 81.4 (2014)*, ZA5928 Data file Version 2.0.0. doi:10.4232/1.12201; *Eurobarometer 82.3 (2014)*, ZA5932 Data file Version 2.0.1. doi:10.4232/1.12259; *Eurobarometer 83.1 (2015)*, ZA5964 Data file Version 1.0.0. doi:10.4232/1.12340; *Eurobarometer 83.3 (2015)*, ZA5998 Data file Version 1.0.0. doi:10.4232/1.12356.

Chapter 10
Analysis of Differences in Trends Among the Satisfied Few and the Dissatisfied Few

Mean Satisfaction in Subgroups of the Population

To this point we have only described how the Reference Distribution can be used to estimate means for an entire population, given that the frequency distributions have been obtained using a discrete verbal scale and a reference distribution for a given year, see Chaps. 8 and 9. While it is important to study the trends in mean for an entire population, in practice scholars are often interested in subgroups of a society which might not be well described by a mean, for example from the perspective of inequality or marginalization. Thus, it would be valuable to be able to break down the distribution found for an entire population at various points.[1] In this section we will show that once a continuous distribution has been found to estimate a population mean for life satisfaction, it is also possible to estimate the mean for subgroups of that population such as the least satisfied and the most satisfied part. In the sections that follow, we will accordingly describe how this method can be extended and used to analysis of trends over time. Using examples from the European Social Survey (ESS) and the Eurobarometer (EB), we will demonstrate this for the topics satisfaction with life and satisfaction with how democracy works in a respondents country. As in Chap. 9 the ESS and EB data on these items was divided into three groups of countries: Western Europe, Southern Europe and Eastern Europe and the example discussed here is based on these groups.

Suppose that the parameters α and β of the estimated beta distribution for life satisfaction in a population are given, then the mean life satisfaction within subgroups of this population can be estimated by making use of the inverse beta distribution.[2] In Tables C.1–C.6 of Appendix C we have given the parameters of

[1]In previous research we have applied the Reference Distribution Method to demonstrate its use in an analysis of trends in happiness and life satisfaction in subgroups of populations that were based on the demographic characteristics sex, age and level of education (DeJonge et al. 2016).

[2]We used the Excel-function beta.inv to calculate the value of the inverse beta distribution.

T. de Jonge et al., *Diversity in Survey Questions on the Same Topic*, Social Indicators Research Series 68, DOI 10.1007/978-3-319-53261-5_10

the beta distributions estimated for the time series on life satisfaction and satisfaction with how democracy works in countries grouped in Western Europe, Southern Europe and Eastern Europe according to the description given in section "Research question". For example, the parameters of the beta distribution estimated for satisfaction with democracy in Southern Europe in the reference year 2012 are: $\alpha = 1.56$ and $\beta = 2.15$. The value of the inverse of this beta distribution for the 25th percentile point is equal to 2.4, meaning that the estimated value of satisfaction with how democracy works is 2.4 or lower for the subgroup of the 25% of people in the population who are least satisfied with how democracy works in their country. In a similar way the inverse of the beta distribution at the 75th percentile point is equal to 5.9, meaning that the value of satisfaction with how democracy works for the subgroup of the 25% of people in the population who are most satisfied with how democracy works in their country is at least 5.9. The inverse beta distributions of the reference distributions derived from the numerical scales of European Social Survey for the frequency distributions of the Eurobarometer in 2012 are shown in Fig. 10.1. We have also depicted four quartile groups in each graph of this figure. The most left of the quartile groups represents the 25% least satisfied people in the population and the most right quartile group represents the 25% most satisfied people.

Clearly, the inverse beta distributions for life satisfaction differ markedly from those for satisfaction with democracy. This is in line with the eye catching differences in cumulative frequency distributions between both topics discussed in Chap. 9, see Fig. 9.3.

Differences in Trends Among the Satisfied Few and the Dissatisfied Few

We calculated the value of the inverse beta distribution for 2.500 equidistant points in each of the quartile groups per topic for all three groups of countries. The average of this large number of values for a quartile group is an estimate of mean life satisfaction or satisfaction with how democracy works in this group in 2012. The estimates of mean life satisfaction in 2012 in Western Europe calculated in this way for the four quartile groups are, for example, respectively 4.4, 6.7, 8.0 and 9.3 and for satisfaction with democracy in Southern Europe to respectively 1.4, 3.2, 4.9 and 7.3.

We estimated the means for each quartile group and both topics for all the Eurobarometer waves in the period 2004–2015, using the beta distributions for each year the parameters of which are presented in Tables C.1–C.6 of Appendix C: for life satisfaction the results of these estimations per quartile group are shown in Fig. 10.2 and for satisfaction with how the democracy works in Fig. 10.3, going counter clockwise from the most satisfied quartile group in the upper right of each figure to the least satisfied quartile group in the lower right. We are aware that the

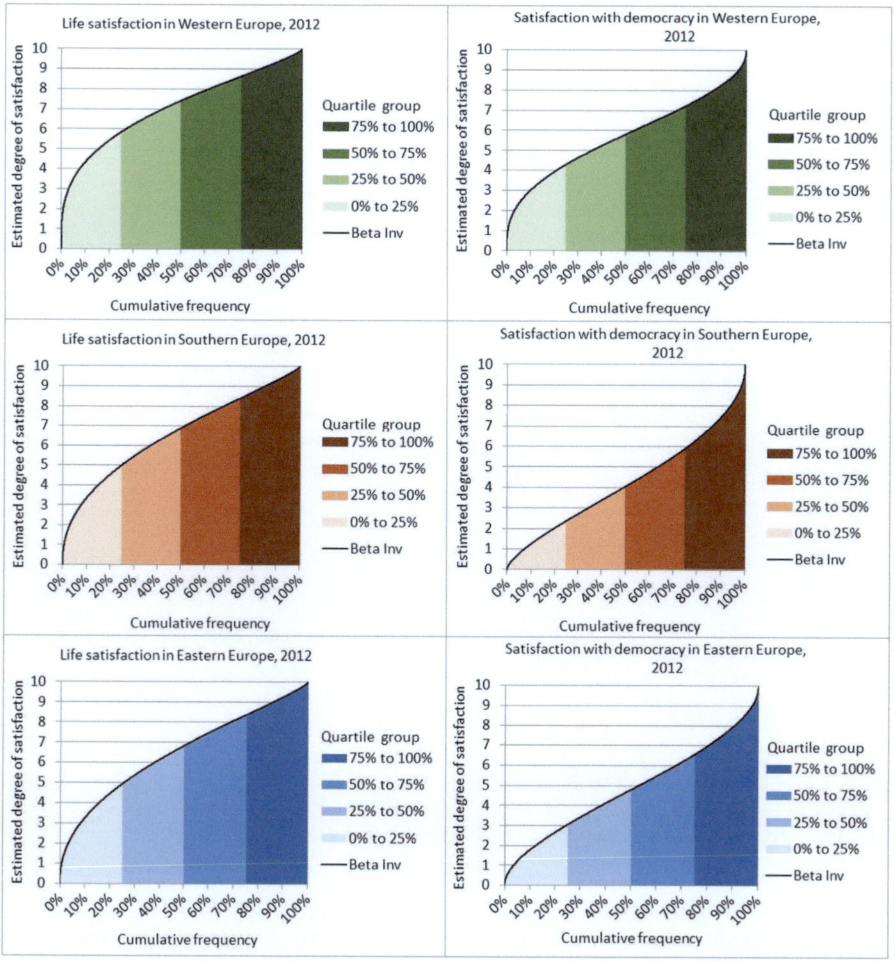

Fig. 10.1 The inverse beta distribution and quartile groups

boundaries between the four response options of the primary scale may be different for each quartile group. From previous research however, we have concluded that the reference boundaries define the levels of the estimated means, but do not influence the evolution of the trends in subgroups (DeJonge et al. 2016, p. 344).

It can be seen from Fig. 10.2 that mean life satisfaction in Western Europe shows a more or less linear upward trend in all of the four quartile groups. Mean life satisfaction in Eastern Europe fluctuates around a constant value for each quartile group, which is, from the most satisfied to the least satisfied quartile group, 9.2, 7.7, 6.0 and 3.5. The largest difference in trends between the quartile groups is apparent in Southern Europe. In the 75–100% quartile group in Southern Europe mean life satisfaction decreased until 2009 when it reached the same level as in Eastern Europe. Since then there the trend in both groups of countries has been

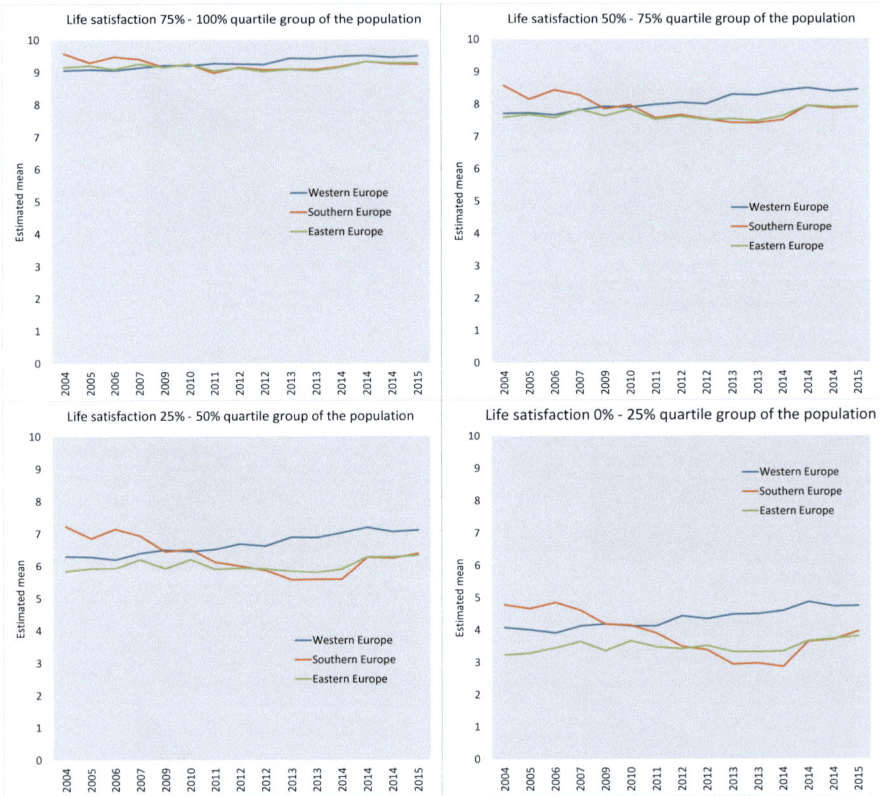

Fig. 10.2 Trends in life satisfaction per quartile group and group of countries

almost similar and nearly stable over time. Something similar can be noticed for the 50–75% quartile group. In the two most dissatisfied quartile groups, mean life satisfaction has decreased to a level below that in Eastern Europe, but in the Southern Europe group in 2014 it increased upwards to the nearly stable level seen in Eastern Europe.

Mean satisfaction with how democracy works in the country shows an increasing trend over time for all quartile groups in Western Europe as can be seen from Fig. 10.3. In Southern Europe the trend is reversed and shows the strongest decrease in estimated mean for the two quartile groups in the middle. For these quartile groups, the gap between the estimated means compared to Western Europe and Eastern Europe in the period from 2010 on, is larger than the gaps for the highest and lowest quartile group.

Where life satisfaction in the two most satisfied quartile groups has not changed much in Southern Europe between 2004 and 2015, this cannot be said for the satisfaction with how democracy works in the country. Satisfaction with how democracy works has decreased rapidly in these two quartile groups and unlike life satisfaction has not kept pace with the trend in Eastern Europe.

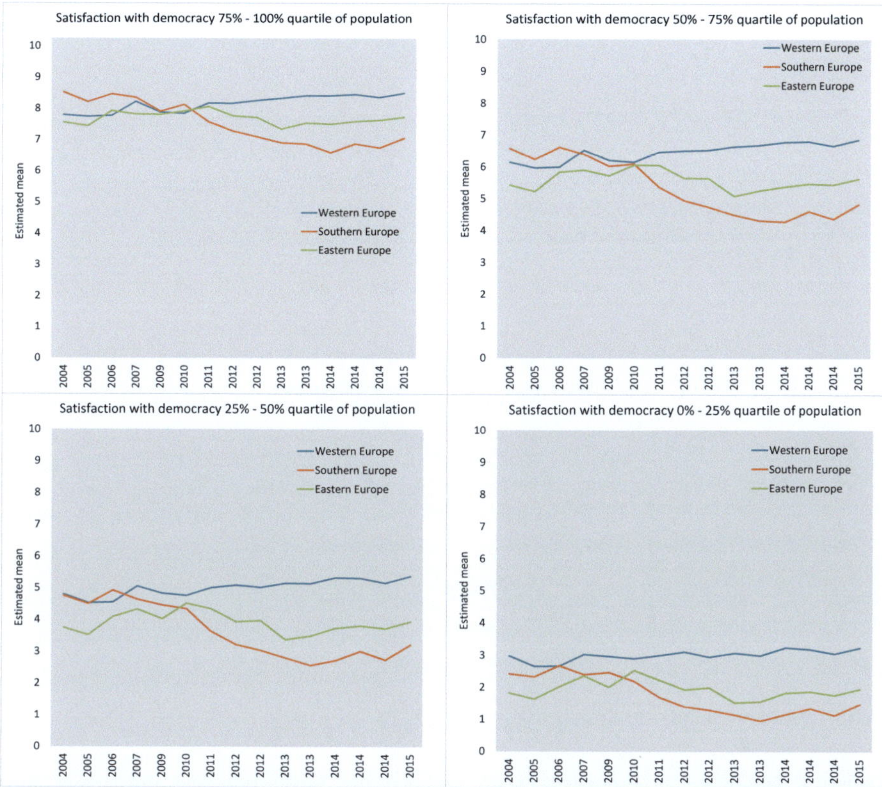

Fig. 10.3 Trends in satisfaction with the democracy per quartile group and group of countries

An impression of the trends in the difference in mean between satisfaction with life and satisfaction with democracy per quartile group for each group of countries is given in Fig. 10.4.

As shown in Figs. 10.2 and 10.3 the trends for the quartile groups in Southern Europe are most marked in Fig. 10.4 showing differences in estimated means between life satisfaction and satisfaction with how democracy works. Once again we can see that the gap between the estimated mean for life satisfaction and satisfaction with how democracy works has become very large in the years that have passed since 2004 for the two middle quartile groups. The trend in mean difference for the lowest quartile group differs remarkably from the trends for the other quartile groups in Southern Europe. This is also the case for the lowest quartile group in Western Europe, for which the gap between the two domains of satisfaction has grown considerably since 2011; in contrast the gap for the other quartile groups has not changed much in the same period.

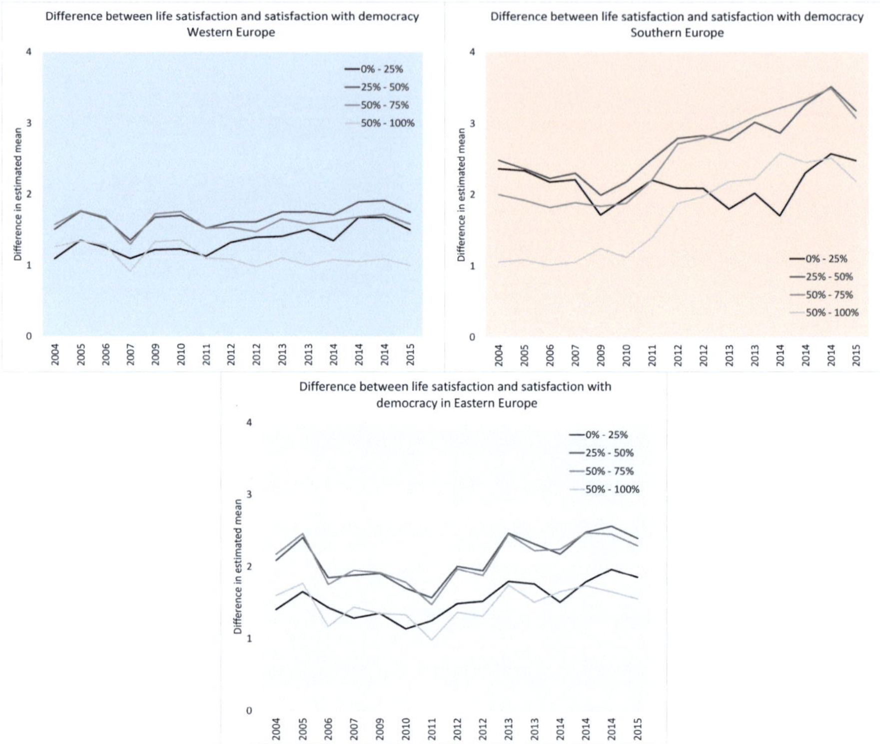

Fig. 10.4 Difference in estimated means between life satisfaction and satisfaction with democracy

Discussion

We have shown that once a continuous distribution is found to estimate the population means for life satisfaction over time, it becomes possible to estimate means for subgroups of a population such as the least satisfied and the most satisfied part. We chose to demonstrate this using quartile groups of populations, but given there is a continuous distribution, means can be estimated for any part of the population. This is not possible when the data to be studied are measured on a discrete scale, as long as the latent distribution underlying such measurements is unknown. Additional research is required to assess the reliability of the estimated means obtained for subgroups using the methodology discussed here. In our opinion, at this point we can say that these means at least give us an indication of the differences in trends between subgroups, which can be useful from the perspective of determining factor of inequality or marginalization in a population.

We are aware that the boundaries between the options of the primary scale may be different for each quartile group, but we believe that there is evidence to support the idea that the reference boundaries define the levels of the estimated means, but do not influence the evolution of the trends in subgroups (DeJonge et al. 2016). More research, however, is necessary to reconfirm this statement.

Reference

DeJonge, T., Veenhoven, R., Moonen, L., Kalmijn, W. M., van Beuningen, J., & Arends, L. R. (2016). Conversion of verbal response scales. Robustness across demographic categories. *Social Indicators Research, 126*, 331–358. doi:10.1007/s11205-015-0897-6.

Chapter 11
Combining and Pooling of Time Series on Life Satisfaction in the USA, Japan, The Netherlands and Spain

Research Question

In Chap. 1 we raised the problem of the incomparability of time series taken from different surveys, and illustrated what the effect is for time series on survey questions about happiness and life satisfaction if the means for both topics are based on just the ranks of response options of the primary scale in Fig. 1.1 of section "The incomparability of time series from different surveys and different time periods". In the earlier parts of this book we discussed a number of conventional and more recently developed approaches to tackle this problem of incomparability, of which the Reference Distribution Method comes closest to overcoming the problem.

The main question we address in this section is: Is the Reference Distribution Method suitable to use for pooling time series based on slightly different survey questions about the same topic? This question has been addressed for time series on life satisfaction and happiness taken from surveys in The Netherlands for a time period of 40 years (DeJonge et al. 2016). This led to the conclusion that in the past 40 years the Dutch have become slightly happier and satisfied with their lives. For this chapter we have gone a step further and have investigated the suitability of using the Reference Distribution Method to pool time series for life satisfaction in the USA, Japan, The Netherlands and Spain, and as a by-product of this investigation, we were able to compare the trends in life satisfaction for these four countries, these trends are also reported and discussed here.

T. de Jonge et al., *Diversity in Survey Questions on the Same Topic*, Social Indicators Research Series 68, DOI 10.1007/978-3-319-53261-5_11

Distortion of Trends Due to Biases in Measurement

A number of sources of measurement bias can be determined which may affect a respondent's response to survey items and muddle the trend analyses by causing discontinuities. Some of these biases can be reduced using the Reference Distribution Method. Therefore a thorough inspection of a time series of data is necessary to determine possible biases that may occur and which have to be addressed before any application of the method to obtain a transformed time series.

In Chap. 5 we introduced the issue of scale effects arising from differences in the numbers of response options, the labeling of the response options and whether a scale is numerical or verbal, however, something we did not mention above, is that the visual presentation of a scale can also influence results. This set of scale effects provided the main motivation and angle of approach for the development of the Reference Distribution Method and the preceding scale transformation methods commonly used in social research. All the methods used to date are aimed at overcoming the incomparability of survey results arousing from the scale effects. Further, if these methods are going to be used to transform time series to perform analyses of trends over a long time span, than a number of other sources of response bias must be addressed. Here we give an overview of these response biases in relation to the Reference Distribution Method. This overview is based on the description of these issues to be found in Stone and Mackie (2013, Chap. 4). In this book the sources of response bias we will deal with are, besides those of scale effects, mode of surveying, ordering of questions, response shift and contextual influences.

Survey Mode Effects

Surveys can be conducted in a number of modes, such as face-to-face, by telephone, paper-and-pencil surveying, via the internet or a mixture of the modes. Which mode is chosen, depends amongst other things on the goal of the survey, the costs of surveying or the size of the sample, and, something which is of importance in relation to time series, the time when, historically, the survey was conducted. Telephone interviews, for example, only became possible after the time it was reasonable that almost all of the respondents would have a telephone at home, however, the rise in mobile phone usage has come at the cost of the adequate registration of telephone numbers, causing this mode of questioning to become statistically invalid. The internet has opened up new opportunities for interviewing and its use is becoming ever more popular for survey research, not in the least for the relatively low costs associated with this mode of surveying.

The mode of surveying used has a large impact on a respondent's response. We mentioned the mode change from computer assisted personal interviews to a paper-and-pencil questionnaire for the Life Situation Survey of SCP (section "Scale transformation using the reference distribution method"), which caused a dramatic fall in the percentage of people who rated themselves as either 'Happy' or 'Very happy'.[1] Another example of the mode effect is described by Dolan and Kavetsos (2012), who found large differences in survey mode which swamped all the other bias effects that they had taken into account in their analysis. Similar findings make Pudney (2010, p. 19) conclude that telephone interviewing may be particularly vulnerable to distortion, because the degree of privacy is unknown and the display of response scales via show cards or computer screens is impossible.

We recall from section "Scale transformation using the reference distribution method" that as long as the mode of surveying is unchanged, the application of the Continuum Approach results for each survey wave in an estimated beta distribution that tightly fits the reference boundaries derived from a reference distribution and the cumulative distribution of the primary scale. If the mode of surveying does not change, the reference boundaries can thus be kept fixed over time and the differences in estimated means can solely be attributed to changes in the frequency distributions on the primary scale.

Ordering of Questions

Stone and Mackie (2013) mention a number of studies in which the effect question ordering has on the response to a survey is discussed. They refer among others to a paper of Deaton (2012), who found a large effect of question ordering on the responses to a question on subjective life satisfaction. How a question was answered, was affected by, for example, whether or not respondents had to answer a question about a subject such as politics or unemployment before they assessed their own satisfaction with life. More in general it is acknowledged in the literature that preceding questions may affect how respondents interpret the meaning of survey items and that this effect may be significantly large (Schwartz and Sudman 1992; OECD 2013; Deaton and Stone 2016).

The bias in trend analyses caused by the effect the question ordering has on the survey response cannot be solved using the Reference Distribution Method if the order of questions is changed in different waves of one and the same survey, unless the size of the effect is comparable to that of a mode change and can be addressed as

[1]This change may be attributed to those responding to a paper-and- pencil survey having more time to think about their answer than someone doing a face-to-face interview, where the pace is set by the interviewer. This leads to a more cognitive than intuitive response which comes with lower reported happiness (Studer and Winkelmann 2014). Another explanation for the change from 2002 to 2004 is the commonly recognized interviewer bias, caused by the effect an interviewer can have on the response in a face-to-face interview (Katz 1942; Davis et al. 2010). The interviewer may, unintentionally, influence respondents to give for example socially desirable answers that may be more positive than when that respondent answers questions in an uninfluenced situation like a paper-and-pencil survey.

such. The Reference Distribution Method however, can deal with a difference in question ordering if this difference is present *between* surveys, but not in succeeding waves of each survey separately. This is because in the Reference Distribution Method the sample means of different surveys are forced to a level that is equivalent to that of the reference distribution, this causing the potential effect of a difference in question ordering between surveys to vanish.

Response Shift

The term 'response shift' originates from a study by Howard et al. (1979) conducted to study to what extent participants changed their level of self-perceived dogmatism during communication skills training. The effect of the training made the participants change their internal standards for their measurement of dogmatism. Researchers introduced the term 'response shift' to denote this kind of change. Since this time a growing number of studies on response shift have been conducted, most in the field of health care (e.g. Schwartz et al. 2013).

Within the field of subjective well-being Stone and Mackie (2013) summarize response shift as a term that is used to characterize changes in reporting over time. They differentiate the observed differences over time in self-reports of well-being into two main streams. One reflects true changes in the quality-of-life assessments made by respondents as a result of adaptation to changed circumstances. The second reflects measurement errors associated with a respondent's internal scale recalibrations. An example of this type of internal scale recalibration, given by Stone and Mackie (2013, p. 76), is the case described of a person with chronic pain who rates this pain on average at 7 on a scale from 1 to 10. After having experienced the more intense pain of a kidney stone, the same person lowered their rating of the unchanged chronic pain to 5. Thus, this person made an internal scale recalibration of how they rate chronic pain.

Stone and Mackie conclude that adaptation cannot be characterized as a process that occurs uniformly, because every person is unique and adapts differently to changing situations. In analyzing time series however, it is of interest to monitor if there are general upwards or downwards trends in target groups or subgroups, and in subjective well-being trends which reflect true changes in quality-of-life, but, as described by Stone and Mackie, it is not yet possible to decompose these trends into what are 'true' changes in quality-of-life and effects of scale recalibration. Use of the Reference Distribution Method does not contribute to solving this entanglement. It is very well possible that over the course of time a slow change in scale interpretation has evolved which means that on average the present population will evaluate the response options in a response scale differently than that of earlier times, which can also be considered as a type of scale recalibration. For an application of the Reference Distribution Method, in which we try to bring sample means from different surveys to a comparable level, we assume that if at present response options are evaluated differently than in the past, this will have been the case for all the response scales under consideration, verbal and numerical.

Contextual Influences

Contextual influences refers to the influence of the research instruments used and the external circumstances at the time of a respondent's assessment for a self-report. The contextual influences of a research instrument can be deconstructed into the mode of surveying used and the ordering of questions, as discussed above. There are manifold influential external circumstances that one can think of, such as the weather conditions at the time of the assessment, recent life events or breaking news of the day, but the demographic characteristics of a respondent, such as age, level of education or cultural background and whether a questionnaire is computer mediated or not can also have an effect on a respondents' answer.

When analyzing trends one has to be aware of these contextual influences. This holds especially when studying trends over a long period of time as a consequence of which the sample of respondents in the earlier waves of the time series represent a different population to that of the present sample of respondents in the more recent waves. In an ageing society for example, an increasing trend in life satisfaction might be due to a positivity effect of an age-related trend of an older person having a positive view towards life (Stone and Mackie 2013). In another example, the composition of a population may change over the years due to immigration and emigration, introducing an effect of changing cultural influences into the outcome of happiness measurements (Senik 2013). The above examples serve to illustrate how contextual influences in general affect trend analyses, independent of the response scales used. The Reference Distribution Method can be used appropriately to take a limited number of the possible contextual influences into account. If, for example, a survey is always conducted in the autumn or spring, than there may be a seasonal effect in the response to each wave, also, when an exceptionally influential event takes places during the period of surveying, for example the 9/11 attacking of the World Trade Center in New York or the FIFA World Cup, the results may be biased. These types of contextual influences are, to a certain extent, corrected when the Reference Distribution Method is used, because the sample means of the surveys they belong to are shifted to a level that is equivalent to that of the reference distribution.

Time Series on Life Satisfaction in the USA, Japan, The Netherlands and Spain

We introduced a number of survey items on life satisfaction from some long running surveys in the USA, Japan and The Netherlands in section "The incompa rability of time series from different surveys and different time periods". In this section we will describe some additional items on life satisfaction used in other surveys in these countries, to complement the set of items we used here to pool time series on life satisfaction. First we will go into some cross-national surveys. The time series used for Spain all come from the cross-national surveys, as do the complementary time series for The Netherlands. The complementary items on life satisfaction are drawn from national surveys in the USA and Japan and will be described below.

Cross-National Surveys The European Values Study (EVS)[2] is a cross-national survey research program on basic human values which started in 1981 with a survey conducted in the European member states. The EVS is repeated every 9 years in a growing number of European countries. The World Values Survey (WVS),[3] which we initially described in section "The continuum approach and discrete numerical scales", is a cross-national survey which builds on the EVS. The first wave of the WVS was conducted in the time frame from 1981 to 1984 in a small number of countries. The second wave followed in the 5 years period from 1990 to 1994 and a new wave for every 5 years period since then has expanded this survey so it is now done in almost 100 countries, and encompasses nearly 90% of the world's population. The trend variables and data from the EVS and the WVS have been harmonized which allowed the construction of an Integrated Values Surveys 1981–2014 the data from which we used for our analyses. In the remainder we will refer to this integrated survey as data from the WVS. The WVS was conducted in all four countries considered in this chapter.

The items on life satisfaction from the Eurobarometer (EB) and the European Social Survey (ESS) were discussed extensively in Chaps. 9 and 10. We will use the time series, based on these items, for The Netherlands and Spain. The time series from the EB span the period from 1973 to 2015 for the Netherlands and from 2002 to 2015 for Spain. The time series extracted from the ESS we have available, covers the period from 2002 to 2014 for The Netherlands and from 2002 to 2012 for Spain.

USA In section "The incomparability of time series from different surveys and different time periods" we only discussed items on life satisfaction taken from the Gallup Poll. Another long running survey in the USA with an item on life satisfaction is the Behavioral Risk Factor Surveillance System (BRFSS).[4] The BRFSS is a

[2]http://www.europeanvaluesstudy.eu/page/integrated-values-surveys-1981-2008.html

[3]http://www.worldvaluessurvey.org/wvs.jsp

[4]http://www.cdc.gov/brfss/

system of health-related telephone surveys used to collect state data about residents from the USA, started in 1984 in 15 states, by 1995 all of the American states were participants. Life satisfaction has been measured in the BRFSS since 2005, with the exceptions of 2011 and 2012, using the question "In general, how satisfied are you with your life?" and a 4-point verbal scale with the response options labeled 'Very satisfied', 'Somewhat satisfied', 'Somewhat dissatisfied' and 'Very dissatisfied'. This same item has also been used in the Latin American Public Opinion Project (LAPOP)[5] in 2008, 2010 and 2012. The origin of LAPOP lies in public opinion research carried out in Costa Rica in the 1970s. Today the project is hosted by the Vanderbilt University in Nashville, Tennessee, today the project regularly carries out public opinion surveys in nearly every country in Latin America, Canada, the United States, and much of the Caribbean.

Japan In addition to the time series using the items from the Life-in-Nation survey (LIN) described in section "The incomparability of time series from different surveys and different time periods", we used time series on life satisfaction from three other surveys conducted in Japan. The first of these is the East Asia Value Survey (EAVS)[6] in which respondents are asked to answer the question "In a word, are you satisfied or dissatisfied with your current life?" and given the options 'Satisfied', 'Somewhat satisfied', 'Neither satisfied nor dissatisfied', 'Somewhat dissatisfied' and 'Dissatisfied' to choose from. The second additional survey is the Lifestyle Preference Survey (LPS)[7] done for the governmental cabinet of Japan. The item on life satisfaction employed in this survey consists of the question "How satisfied or dissatisfied are you with your life in general?" and the response options 'Satisfied', "Somewhat satisfied', 'Neither satisfied nor dissatisfied', 'Rather dissatisfied' and 'Dissatisfied'. The third additional item is taken from the Future Life Survey (FLS), which consists of the question "How satisfied are you with your current life as a whole?" and the response options 'Satisfied', 'Fairly satisfied', 'Neither satisfied nor dissatisfied', 'Somewhat dissatisfied' and 'Dissatisfied'.

An overview of the cumulative frequency distributions per year of the time series we have used in this chapter are given in Appendix E. The time series of the mean values per country were obtained using the Rank Method and are shown in Fig. 11.1.

Looking at Fig. 11.1 it is obvious that a comparison across surveys and across countries is difficult when the Rank Method is used.

[5]http://www.vanderbilt.edu/lapop/

[6]http://www.ism.ac.jp/~yoshino/sr/

[7]http://www5.cao.go.jp/seikatsu/senkoudo/senkoudo.html

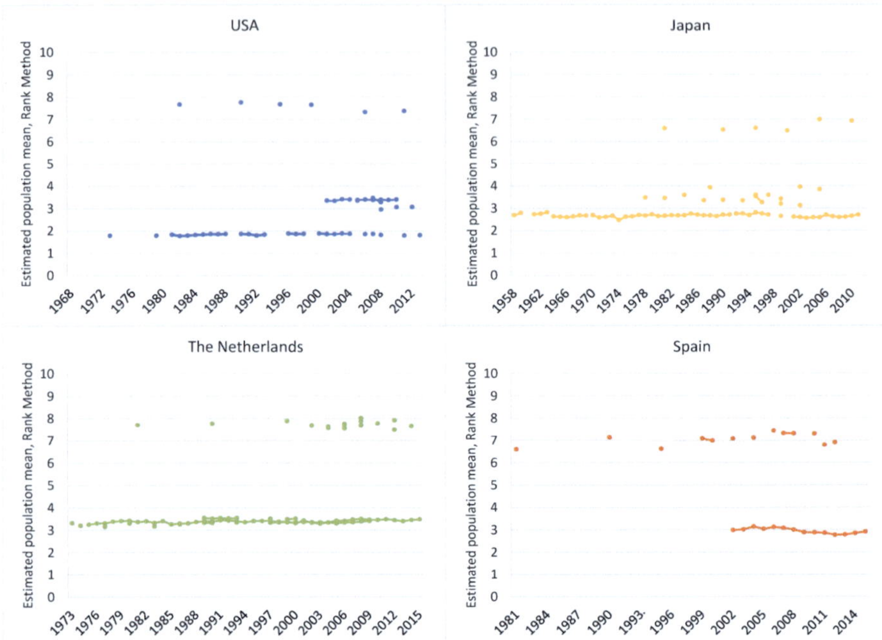

Fig. 11.1 Time series of mean life satisfaction based on the Rank Method

Searching for Sources for Response Bias to Correct

We have argued that using the Reference Distribution Method makes it possible to correct for discontinuities due to mode changes and, to a limited extent, for contextual influences. To do this requires a thorough inspection of the available time series, and decisions have to be made as to which waves require new reference boundaries to be derived and which of the estimated beta distributions can serve as a reference for these decisions. In addition we have to decide whether some waves have to be excluded from a transformation and for what valid reason.

The USA The life satisfaction item in the Gallup Poll in the period from 1973 to 2001 uses a 2-point verbal scale. Unfortunately, we cannot use this item when applying the Reference Distribution Method, since, as we remarked in section "An impression of the diversity in survey items", the number of perfectly fit beta distributions for a 2-point scale is infinite, and use of the Continuum Approach is therefore invalidated, for the same reason, we cannot use the 2-point verbal scale item Gallup introduced in 2001. For the BRFSS, due to a change in the weighting methodology and the addition of a cell phone sampling frame, the data of the 2013 and 2014 waves are not directly comparable with results from earlier waves. Since we have no data from other surveys for 2013 or 2014, we decided not to make use of the BRFSS waves for these years. Further, the mode applied in the WVS was changed from face-to-face interviews to internet surveying in the 2006 wave. The previous wave of the WVS was conducted in 1999 in the USA. We did not correct for this mode change in the WVS, as there was a gap of 2 years between 1999 and the next year life satisfaction was measured in the USA.

Japan We are not aware of any mode changes applied to the Japanese surveys, except for a change from face-to-face interviewing to paper-and-pencil surveying in the WVS. According to the documentation of the WVS, this change took place in the fourth wave which was conducted in 2000. When we look at the frequency distributions of the WVS in Table E.2.8, however, a clear discontinuity can be noted between the 2000 and the 2005 wave and not between the 1995 and 2000 wave. We therefore corrected for the discontinuity observed in the transition from 2000 to 2005.

The Netherlands The surveys of CBS and SCP which include the verbal scale item on life satisfaction have been changed several times since their introduction. These changes have affected the responses and led to serious discontinuities in the time series. In the first years the survey containing the item was only fielded over a period of a few weeks per year, changing to a continuous survey from 1989 on. A comprehensive revision of the questionnaire forms and a reduction in the number of survey items in several domains in 1994 led once more to a response discontinuity. Another major change in the CBS survey took place in 1997 when among other things the survey mode was changed from paper-and-pencil surveying into face-to-face interviews. This change was introduced using a split-half measurement with half of the respondents being required to fill in a paper-and-pencil questionnaire and the other half being interviewed. CBS changed to a mix-mode of surveying in 2010 which caused a drop of approximately 5% in the percentage of satisfied persons, so for this reason we left the results for 2010 out of the conversion process. In the most recent change to the CBS survey, in 2012, 10-point numerical scales were introduced, breaking with the previous tradition of using verbal scales (Van Beuningen et al. 2014). We also left the 2012 wave of CBS out of the conversion process, since, due to the previous comment, as yet it provides only a singular point in the CBS data flow. Much of which has been said for the CBS items also holds for the SCP items. In addition, for rating life satisfaction SCP changed from using its traditional 5-point verbal scale to a 10-point numerical scale in 2004.

The mode applied in the WVS was changed from face-to-face interviews to CAPI[8] in the wave conducted in 2006. We did not find it necessary to correct for this mode change, because we did not see a remarkable change in the response pattern that could be attributed to the mode change.

Spain The mode of surveying with the WVS changed from face-to-face interviewing to CAPI in Spain in 2008, just as for The Netherlands, we had no reason to correct for this change.

[8]CAPI = Computer Assisted Personal Interviewing.

Eurobarometer In the waves of the EB from before 2002 the questions on life satisfaction, were preceded by a number of opinion questions on different topics. In almost all waves of the EB from 2002 on, the question on life satisfaction is the first subjective question asked. We have seen no noticeable change due to this difference in question ordering between older and newer waves. The main point of concern with respect to the EB is the fact that there is a spring and a summer wave in each year and in some years one or more extra waves. This may be the reason why the individual waves of the time series of the EB show a rather irregular pattern, which may be due to seasonal effects. For this reason, but also because we preferred to have one measurement a year, we averaged the response to all waves per year for the EB for The Netherlands and for Spain.

Preparation for the Conversion of Time Series

The WVS is the only survey available in which life satisfaction is measured on a 10-point numerical scale and which is fielded in all of the four countries of interest. The WVS is therefore an obvious choice to select when estimating initial reference distributions. Except for the Japanese waves from before 2005, which we needed to correct for the previously mentioned mode change, we estimated a best fit beta distribution to the frequency distributions of each wave of the WVS in each of the four countries, keeping the numerical response options equidistant. In this way we got a conversion of the time series from the WVS into a series of continuous distributions fitting the 0–10 continuum.

The best fitting beta distributions based on measurements by the WVS during the period of the fifth wave from 2005 to 2009 were used as reference distributions for our application of the Reference Distribution Method. For the USA the reference distribution was based on the measurement done in 2007 and for Japan on the response of 2005. In The Netherlands and Spain, however, life satisfaction was measured in the WVS in the period from 2005 to 2009, and in the European Values Survey (EVS) in 2006 and 2008, and, since the data on life satisfaction from the EVS and the WVS have been harmonized, see section "Time series on life satisfaction in the USA, Japan, The Netherlands and Spain", we choose to use the best fit beta distribution based on the EVS data as reference distributions for The Netherlands and Spain. The reason for this choice is that the number of other surveys measuring life satisfaction in the years the EVS was fielded was larger than for the years in which the WVS was fielded in The Netherlands and Spain.

A problem that we recognize, but will not deal with in this book, is that the mode of surveying of the WVS in the years which we used to base the initial reference distributions on are not the same for all the countries. The mode used in The Netherlands and Spain is CAPI, the USA measured life satisfaction using internet surveying, in Japan a paper-and-pencil questionnaire was send by postal mail to the respondents. Here we will concentrate on across survey comparability and accept that for now the across country comparability after conversion of the time series will not be as appropriate as we would like it to be. We will discuss this further at the end of this chapter.

Having found the reference distribution for each country, we made a conversion scheme for each country to serve as an aid to prepare and support the conversion process. The scheme for the USA is the smallest of the four schemes and is shown in Fig. 11.2. In this scheme the waves of the WVS item are indicated by the corresponding year on the left side. It can be seen from Fig. 11.2 that several conversion rounds are needed for the conversion process. This is a consequence of the fact that not all the surveys were in use for the entire period spanned by all the time series together. The dark coloured boxes with text in white in Fig. 11.2 represent a year and survey item for which a beta distribution is estimated which is used to derive reference boundaries from for other survey items. The reference boundaries derived for each of those other surveys on their turn are used to apply the Continuum Approach for estimating a best fit beta distribution for each of the other waves in the corresponding column. This is indicated, for example, for the waves of the BRFSS item in the period 2005–2010 by the text '2006' in Fig. 11.2.

From Fig. 11.2 it can be seen that we needed to derive reference boundaries for a number of items and a number of years. The reference boundaries for the 2004 wave of the Gallup item O-SLP-c-sq-v-4-a were derived from the estimated beta distribution for the 2005 wave of the Gallup item O-SLu-u-sq-v-4-f, which means that there was a 1 year difference between the waves from both surveys. This was a choice we made, because otherwise we would not have been able to convert the time series for this Gallup item. The vertical bar in the scheme of Fig. 11.2 is used to indicate that we do have measurements for all years in between the year on the left preceding this bar and the year succeeding the bar.

We have presented the reference boundaries we derived in each round of the conversion process for life satisfaction in Table 11.1, including the parameters α and β and the estimated population mean for each reference distribution used.

It can be seen from Table 11.1 that although all the items have the same response options, the reference boundaries between these options are different. This corroborates with the idea that how a response option with a certain label is interpreted depend on the context of the scale, see Chap. 5.

The conversion scheme for Japan is given in Fig. 11.3, from which it is clear that five conversion rounds are needed. The conversion of the waves of the WVS is divided over two rounds. In the first round best beta distributions are estimated for the Japanese WVS waves of 2005 and 2012, for which the boundaries between the response options are assumed to be equally distanced. In the second round, best fit beta distributions for the older waves were estimated, based on the reference distribution derived from the beta distributions that best fits the 1995 wave of the LIN item O-SLW-c-sq-v-4-e. For the conversion of the times series based on the LIN item used in the period 1970–1991 is converted in the third round, the beta distribution that best fits the cumulative frequency distribution of the LPS item in the 1990 wave is used as a reference distribution. The time series that need to be converted in the fourth and fifth round show a 1 year difference from the wave from which the reference distribution is derived. We do not have a better solution for this

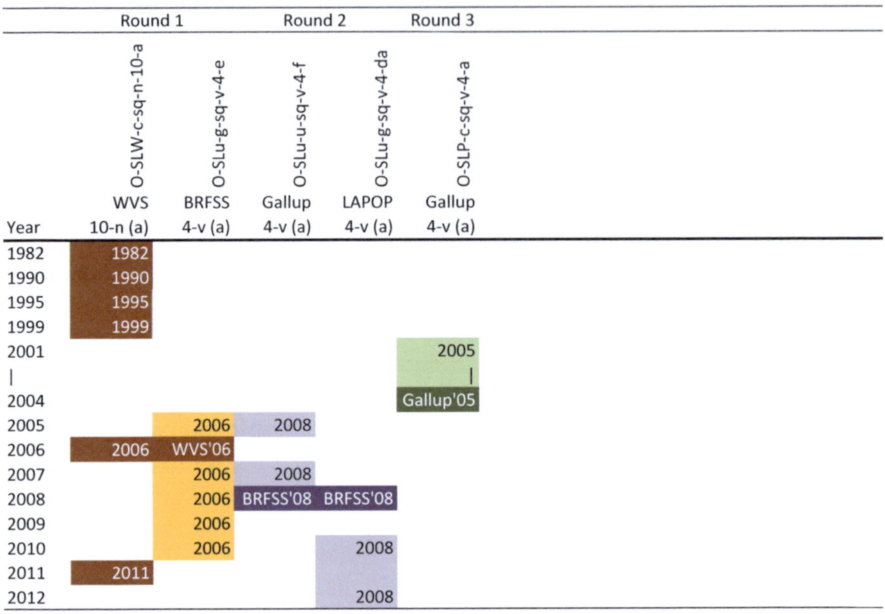

Fig. 11.2 Conversion scheme for life satisfaction in the USA

problem, since we lack data for overlapping years for these time series based on LIN items used in Japan.

The five rounds for the conversion of time series on life satisfaction in Japan leave us with a total of eight sets of reference boundaries, two in the first round, three in the second round and one of each of the other rounds. The parameters and means of the beta distributions from which these reference boundaries have been derived are given in Tables 11.2 and 11.3, followed by the reference boundary for each corresponding response option. The large number of different labels used for the response options used over time to express the degree of life satisfaction is especially striking.

The response options of the WVS scale are assumed to be equidistant for the initial reference distribution based on the WVS wave of 2005. From Tables 11.2 and 11.3 it is clear that this equidistance assumption is no longer valid after correction for the mode change between the 1995 wave and the 2000 wave. The distance between the boundaries of the response options in the lower end of the WVS scale derived on basis of the 1995 wave, reflect the skewness of the frequency distribution.

Although the number of different survey items used to measure life satisfaction in The Netherlands is small, the number of different sets of reference boundaries to be determined is rather large, due to the many mode changes found in the Dutch surveys. This can be seen in Fig. 11.4.

The time series for the EB item and the item used by CBS and SCP span almost the same period of time. Therefore only two conversion rounds were needed for the

Table 11.1 Reference distributions and reference boundaries for the USA

	Round 1	Round 2		Round 3
Reference distribution	WVS 2006	BRFSS 2008		Gallup 2005
	O-SLW-c-sq-n-10-a	O-SLu-g-sq-v-4-e		O-SLu-u-sq-v-4-f
Estimated alpha	4.52	4.44		4.72
Estimated beta	2.14	2.12		2.09
Estimated mean	6.79	6.77		6.93
Response option	BRFSS	Gallup	LAPOP	Gallup
	O-SLu-g-sq-v-4-e	O-SLu-u-sq-v-4-f	O-SLu-g-sq-v-4-da	O-SLP-c-sq-v-4-a
Very satisfied	10.0	10.0	10.0	10.0
Somewhat satisfied	7.17	7.12	8.03	6.70
Somewhat dissatisfied	3.17	4.76	5.57	5.05
Very dissatisfied	2.49	3.63	3.86	3.92

	Round 1			Round 2			Round 3	Round 4	Round 5
	O-SLW-c-sq-n-10-a	O-SLW-c-sq-v-4-e	O-SLu-c-sq-v-5-n	O-SLu-g-sq-v-5-e	O-SLW-c-sq-v-5-k	O-SLW-c-sq-n-10-a	O-SLu-c-sq-v-4-e	O-SLu-u-sq-v-4-e	O-SLu-c-sq-v-4-f
Year	WVS 10-n (a)	LIN 4-v (c)	EAVS 5-v	LPS 5-v (b)	FLS 5-v	WVS 10-n (a)	LIN 4-v (a)	LIN 4-v (b)	LIN 4-v (a)
1958									1964
1959									1964
1961									1964
1962									1964
1963									LIN '64
1964								1970	
1965								1970	
1966								1970	
1967								1970	
1968								1970	
1969								EPA '70	
1970							1990		
1971							1990		
1972							1990		
1973							1990		
1974							1990		
1975							1990		
1976							1990		
1977							1990		
1978				2002			1990		
1979							1990		
1980							1990		
1981				2002			1990		
1982							1990		
1983							1990		
1984				2002			1990		
1985						1995	1990		
1986							1990		
1987				2002			1990		
1988			2005				1990		
1989							1990		
1990				2002		1995	EPA '90		
1991							1990		
1992		2005							
1993		2005		2002					
1994		2005							
1995		2005		2002	1999	LIN 1995			
1996		2005		2002					
1997		2005			1999				
1998									
1999		2005		2002	EPA'99				
2000						1995			
2001		2005							
2002		2005	2005	EPA'02					
2003		2005							
2004		2005							
2005	2005	WVS'05	WVS'05						
2006		2005							
2007		2005							
2008		2005							
2009		2005							
2010		2005							
2011		2005							
2012	2012								

Fig. 11.3 Conversion scheme for life satisfaction in Japan

Table 11.2 Reference distributions and reference boundaries for Japan, round 1 and round 2

	Round 1		Round 2		
	WVS 2005 O-SLW-c-sq-n-10-a		LIN 2002	LIN 1999	LIN 1995
Reference distribution			O-SLW-c-sq-v-4-e		
Estimated alpha		3.97	3.94	3.83	5.36
Estimated beta		2.19	2.16	1.99	2.31
Estimated mean		6.44	6.47	6.58	6.98
Response option	LIN O-SLW-c-sq-v-4-e	EAVS O-SLu-c-sq-v-5-n	LPS O-SLu-g-sq-v-5-e	FLS O-SLW-c-sq-v-5-k	WVS O-SLW-c-sq-n-10-a
Very satisfied					
Satisfied	10.0	10.0	10.0	10.0	
Somewhat satisfied		7.70	9.13		
Fairly satisfied	8.84			9.07	
Neutral		5.48	7.06	6.54	
Somewhat dissatisfied	6.02	4.13		4.66	
Dissatisfied	4.04	2.78	3.60	2.98	
10 Satisfied					10.0
9					9.19
8					8.74
7					7.70
6					6.98
5					6.00
4					4.94
3					4.43
2					3.74
1 Dissatisfied					3.24

conversion process. In the first round, all the reference boundaries can be derived from the beta distribution that best fits the 2006 frequency distribution of the WVS. To derive the reference boundaries for the CBS and SCP time series which include the year 1997, we could choose from the beta distributions that best fits the EB wave in 1997 or the CBS wave in 1997. Obviously, we have chosen the latter option, since the CBS wave of 1997 used in the first round is the same as the CBS and SCP items used in 1997 in the second round. The only difference between the two rounds is the mode of surveying. The parameters and means of the beta distributions from which the reference boundaries for the Dutch time series was derived are given in Tables 11.4 and 11.5.

Similar to what we saw for the Japanese time series measured on a numerical scale, the reference boundaries for the 10-point numerical scale item of SCP and the 11-point numerical scale item of ESS are not equidistance. Looking at Tables 11.4 and 11.5 it can be seen that again for these 2 scales the reference boundaries reflect the skewness of the distribution. Eight different sets of reference boundaries have been derived for the 5-point verbal scale item in Tables 11.4 and 11.5 due to the

Table 11.3 Reference distributions and reference boundaries for Japan, round 3 to 5

	Round 3	Round 4	Round 5
Reference distribution	LPS 1990 O-SLu-g-sq-v-5-e	LIN 1970 O-Slu-c-sq-v-4-e	LIN 1964 O-SLu-u-sq-v-4-e
Estimated alpha	3.81	4.04	4.37
Estimated beta	1.69	1.84	2.08
Estimated mean	6.92	6.87	6.78
Response option	LIN O-SLu-c-sq-v-4-e	LIN O-SLu-u-sq-v-4-e	LIN O-SLu-c-sq-v-4-f
Very satisfied	10.0		
Sufficiently satisfied		10.0	
Life could be better, but on the whole satisfied			10.0
Rather satisfied, but not sufficiently		9.30	
Somewhat satisfied	9.29		
Not satisfied with current life, but not too bad.			8.39
Fairly dissatisfied		6.34	
Somewhat dissatisfied	6.21		
Very dissatisfied	3.43		
My current life is far from satisfactory			6.10
I cannot stand my current life			3.67
Extremely dissatisfied		3.41	

mode changes that have been introduced over time in the Dutch series and the two different surveys using this item. The reference boundaries do differ between the sets, but for a given response option not exceptionally.

Since we did not notice any mode changes in the surveys fielded in Spain and because no more than three different survey items for measuring life satisfaction were used, the conversion scheme for Spain was the most simple and smallest of all the countries. This scheme is given in Fig. 11.5.

The parameters and means of the beta distributions from which the reference boundaries for the Spanish time series have been derived are given in Table 11.6.

The frequency distribution for life satisfaction in Spain is less skewed to the right than in the Netherlands. This is reflected in the values of the reference boundaries, which in the lower parts of the same scales are lower for Spain than for The Netherlands.

Combining Converted Survey Results into Long Time Series

Having prepared the data using the described methods, the data is now ready for the conversion process, the time series of the different survey items for life satisfaction in the four countries can be converted such that the resulting estimated population

	Round 1					Round 2						
	O-SLW-c-sq-n-10-a	O-SLL-u-sq-v-4-b	O-SLL-c-sq-v-5-d	O-SLL-c-sq-n-10-a	O-SLW-c-sq-n-11-cd	O-SLL-c-sq-v-5-d	O-SLL-c-sq-v-5-d	O-SLL-c-sq-v-5-d	O-SLL-c-sq-v-5-d	O-SLL-c-sq-v-5-d	O-SLL-c-sq-v-5-d	O-SLL-c-sq-v-5-d
	WVS	EB	CBS	SCP	ESS	SCP	CBS	CBS	SCP	CBS	CBS	SCP
Year	10p-n	4p-v	5p-v	10p-n	11p-n	5p-v	5p-v	5p-v	5p-v	5p-v	5p-v	5p-v
1973		2006										
1974											1977	1977
1975		2006										
1976		2006										
1977		2006									EB'77	EB'77
1978		2006										
1979		2006										
1980		2006								1986		
1981	1981	2006										
1982		2006										
1983		2006								1986		
1984		2006										
1985		2006										
1986		2006								EB'86		
1987		2006										
1988		2006										
1989		2006						1993	1993			
1990	1990	2006						1993	1993			
1991		2006						1993				
1992		2006						1993				
1993		2006						EB'93	EB'93			
1994		2006					1997					
1995		2006					1997					
1996							1997					
1997		2006	2006			CBS'97	CBS'97					
1998		2006	2006									
1999	1999	2006	2006			1997						
2000		2006	2006			1997						
2001		2006	2006									
2002		2006	2006		2006							
2003		2006	2006									
2004		2006	2006	2006	2006							
2005		2006	2006									
2006	2006	WVS'06	WVS'06	WVS'06	WVS'06							
2007		2006	2006									
2008	2008	2006	2006	2006	2006							
2009		2006	2006									
2010		2006			2006							
2011		2006										
2012	2012	2006			2006							
2013		2006										
2014		2006			2006							
2015		2006										

Fig. 11.4 Conversion scheme for life satisfaction in The Netherlands

means are on a comparable level. Once this is achieved, the converted times series can be pooled into long, consistent, times series for life satisfaction.

Conversion of Population Means for Time Series of Individual Survey Items

Given the estimates of the parameters α and β of the beta distribution of life satisfaction, we can calculate an estimate of the population mean as $10*\alpha/(\alpha + \beta)$ for each survey in a time series, doing this for all the estimated beta distributions, gives a time series of converted population means for each individual survey item.

Table 11.4 Reference distributions and reference boundaries for The Netherlands, round 1

	Round 1			
	WVS 2006 O-SLW-c-sq-n-10-a			
Reference distribution				
Estimated alpha			7.64	
Estimated beta			2.90	
Estimated mean			7.25	
Response option	EB O-SLL-u-sq-v-4-b	CBS O-SLL-c-sq-v-5-d	SCP O-SLL-c-sq-n-10-a	ESS O-SLW-c-sq-n-11-cd
Extraordinarily satisfied		10.0		
Very satisfied	10.0	8.97		
Satisfied		7.69		
Fairly Satisfied	7.49	5.64		
Not very satisfied	4.84	4.55		
Not at all satisfied	3.83			
10 Completely satisfied			10.0	
10 Extremely satisfied				10.0
9			8.97	9.05
8			8.35	8.35
7			6.93	6.97
6			5.68	5.85
5			4.86	5.35
4			4.24	4.84
3			3.98	4.49
2			3.59	3.99
1				3.51
1 Completely dissatisfied			3.31	
0 Extremely dissatisfied				3.27

We recall from section "Scale transformation using the reference distribution method" that if the mode of surveying has not changed, the reference boundaries can be kept fixed over time when applying the Continuum Approach and the differences in estimated means can be attributed solely to changes in the frequency distributions on the primary scale. The use of reference distributions brings the means for different survey items to a comparable level. The time series of the converted means for our four countries are presented in Fig. 11.6. The values of the means follow from the parameters of the beta distributions which are given in Appendix E.

Comparing the converted time series given in Fig. 11.6 with the unconverted time series in Fig. 11.1 it can be seen that the conversion process, as intended, brought the estimated population means to a comparable level, also, the pattern over the year for each individual time series remains largely unchanged after the conversion, except for the waves for which we corrected for discontinuities and for

Table 11.5 Reference distributions and reference boundaries for The Netherlands, round 2

	Round 2						
	CBS 1997			EB 1993	EB 1986	EB 1977	
Reference distribution	O-SLL-c-sq-v-5-d			O-SLL-u-sq-v-4-b			
Estimated alpha	7.58			7.22	7.51	6.88	
Estimated beta	2.90			2.82	3.32	2.94	
Estimated mean	7.23			7.19	6.94	7.01	
Response option	SCP O-SLL-c-sq-v-5-d	CBS O-SLL-c-sq-v-5-d	CBS O-SLL-c-sq-v-5-d	SCP O-SLL-c-sq-v-5-d	CBS O-SLL-c-sq-v-5-d	CBS O-SLL-c-sq-v-5-d	SCP O-SLL-c-sq-v-5-d
Extraordinarily satisfied	10.0	10.0	10.0	10.0	10.0	10.0	10.0
Very satisfied	8.95	8.73	8.61	8.63	8.69	8.81	8.80
Satisfied	7.68	7.40	7.21	7.26	7.45	7.71	7.69
Fairly Satisfied	5.69	5.74	5.50	5.55	5.60	5.84	5.79
Not very satisfied	4.56	4.85	4.49	4.52	4.50	4.74	4.70

	Round 1		
Year	O-SLW-c-sq-n-10-a WVS 10p-n	O-SLL-u-sq-v-4-b EB 4p-v	O-SLW-c-sq-n-11-cd ESS 11p-n
1981	1981		
1990	1990		
1995	1995		
1999	1999		
2000	2000		
2002		2008	2008
2003		2008	
2004		2008	2008
2005		2008	
2006		2008	2008
2007	2007	2008	
2008	2008	WVS'08	WVS'08
2009		2008	
2010		2008	2008
2011	2011	2008	
2012		2008	2008
2014		2008	
2015		2008	

Fig. 11.5 Conversion scheme for life satisfaction in Spain

Table 11.6 Reference distributions and reference boundaries for Spain

	Round 1	
Reference distribution	WVS 2008	
	O-SLW-c-sq-n-10-a	
Estimated alpha	4.02	
Estimated beta	1.91	
Estimated mean	6.78	
Response option	EB	ESS
	O-SLL-u-sq-v-4-b	O-SLW-c-sq-n-11-cd
Very satisfied	10.0	
Fairly satisfied	8.54	
Not very satisfied	4.87	
Not at all satisfied	2.67	
10 Extremely satisfied		10.0
9		8.98
8		8.26
7		6.81
6		5.62
5		4.92
4		3.96
3		3.26
2		2.56
1		2.01
0 Extremely dissatisfied		1.73

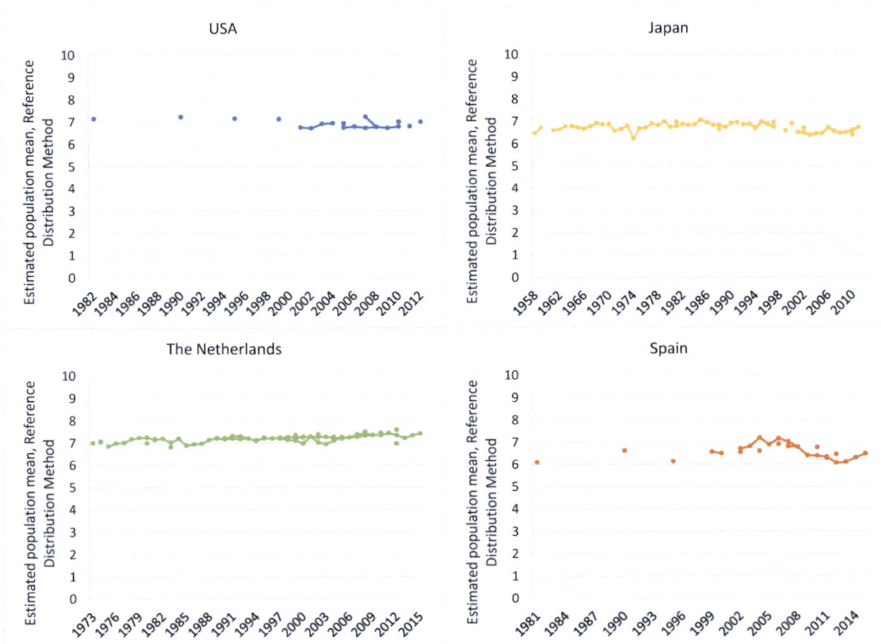

Fig. 11.6 Converted time series of mean life satisfaction for individual survey items

the magnitude of the fluctuations. The magnitude of the fluctuations is a little stretched, due to the conversion of the data from a low number of response options to a continuum spanning a larger numerical range.

Pooling of Converted Time Series

The last step required to obtain one long time series for happiness and life satisfaction is to pool the converted times series of the individual survey items. We choose to pool the time series in the most straightforward manner one can think of, which corresponds to taking the average of the estimated population means for each year. This gives one un-weighted average population mean per year, melding all individual converted time series into the required time series. These pooled time series are shown in Fig. 11.7.

It can be seen from Fig. 11.7 that pooling the converted time series has flattened the fluctuations of the individual time series. We can conclude that mean life satisfaction in Japan and The Netherlands was almost equal in the eighties, but at present differs more than one point in favor of The Netherlands. Mean life satisfaction in the USA moves in between mean life satisfaction in Japan and the Netherlands, and mean life satisfaction in Spain reached its lowest value at 6.0 in 2012, but has increased since then to 6.3 in 2015.

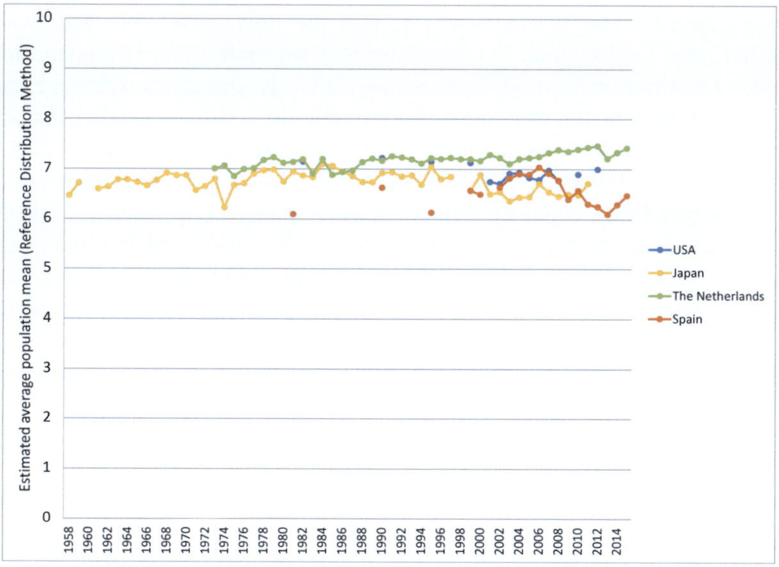

Fig. 11.7 Pooled converted time series for life satisfaction in four countries

Discussion

In this chapter we have presented an example application of the Reference Distribution Method for pooling time series based on slightly different survey questions on the same topic. We used the method to pool time series for satisfaction with life in the USA, Japan, The Netherlands and Spain. In this section we will discuss some methodological considerations.

As we stated in section "Illustration of applying the reference distribution method" the Reference Distribution Method is an attempt to deal with the assumption that, for a given year and a given population, one can expect the estimated distribution means for similar questions about happiness asked in different representative surveys to be approximately the same irrespective of the primary response scales used. This equality of distribution means implies that the estimated cumulative distribution functions are exactly the same for both primary scales, but will lead to different reference boundaries for these primary scales. This requires that the reference distribution must be based on a model which does not depend on the scale of measurement. Beta distributions meet this requirement.

We recall from section "Preparation for the conversion of time series" that the mode of surveying of the WVS in the years which we used to base the initial reference distributions on, are not the same in all of the countries. Although with the Reference Distribution Method a step is made towards improving the across survey comparability for a given topic of interest, these differences in modes hamper the across nation comparability, since the mode of surveying does influence the response patterns. The WVS, however, was the only survey we had available which had been fielded in all our countries and appropriate for demonstrating the Reference Distribution Method. Furthermore, if we assume that a reference value is mainly a determinant for bringing survey results to a certain level, but does not affect the pattern of the trend of a time series (DeJonge et al. 2016), than at least the trends of the pooled time series for the different countries can be compared. Cross national comparability could be improved when using the Reference Distribution Method, if use could be made of a cross country survey from which initial reference distribution could be derived. Such a survey would need to be corrected for biases due to differences in culture and language. The advantage of the Reference Distribution Method is that this type of correction is only required for the cross country survey that is used for the initial reference distribution and not for the other surveys time series that are combined into longer time series.

The standard version of the Eurobarometer has a spring wave and an autumn wave and sometimes one or more extra waves in a year. For the pooling of time series as described in this book, we calculated the un-weighted average of the frequency distributions for each year of the EB, to obtain one sample mean per year. Another option would have been to consider the spring waves and the autumn waves as each constituting different time series and then to convert them separately. In this case, the possible seasonal effect would not have been averaged out before the application of the Reference Distribution Method, but after the conversion when pooling with other survey time series to form one long time series. It would then be possible to investigate whether or not a seasonal effect is more or less stable over time.

There are sizeable differences in the number of respondents per survey to the survey items we looked at. When pooling the converted time series, we did not take these differences into consideration and calculated an un-weighted average for each year. It would be interesting to investigate if the trends found would differ very much if, when averaging over the estimated means in a year, these means were weighted by the number of respondents to the corresponding survey.

We only used one wave of the WVS to estimate an initial reference distribution for the conversion of the time series of one survey. The initial reference distribution defines the level of reference for the conversion results of all waves from each survey. To obtain a more stable pooled time series that is less prone to systematic errors, it would be useful to consider repeating the whole conversion process using each wave of the WVS once to derive an initial reference distribution from for the survey items for which this is possible. Instead of pooling time series which are converted on the basis of just one initial reference distribution, conversion results for initial reference distributions based on other waves could be included in the pooling.

We kept the boundaries between response options that were derived from a reference distribution fixed for all subsequent waves for which the survey design had not undergone a significant change. It is a reasonable assumption that the boundaries will be more or less stable over time and may be kept fixed, as we have described in Chap. 9 and in DeJonge et al. (2015).

The Reference Distribution Method can be used to correct for discontinuities due to mode changes and, to a limited extent, to account for contextual influences; yet, as we already stated in section "Limitations", its use cannot solve all the comparability problems. For example an effect on the response due to a re-ordering of questions cannot be corrected for by the Reference Distribution Method if the effect is small or the re-ordering occurs frequently and affects the responses of a number of waves. Furthermore, if there is a response shift, this will be difficult to correct for since in time series this shift may occur over a long period of time and we assume that if it occurs, this will be the case for all response scales under consideration, both verbal and numerical.

Conclusion

We conclude that the Reference Distribution Method is a useful method to pool time series from different surveys to make the analyses of trends over a long time span possible. Having applied this method to pool time series of responses to different survey items on life satisfaction, we conclude that mean life satisfaction in Japan and The Netherlands was almost equal in the eighties, but at present differs more than one point in favor of The Netherlands. Mean life satisfaction in the USA moves in between mean life satisfaction in Japan and the Netherlands, and mean life satisfaction in Spain reached its lowest value at 6.0 in 2012, but has increased since then to 6.3 in 2015.

References

Davis, R. E., Couper, M. P., Janz, N. K., Caldwell, C. H., & Resnicow, K. (2010). Interviewer effects in public health surveys. *Health Education Research, 25*(1), 14–26., Oxford University Press, doi:10.1093-her-cyp046

Deaton, A. (2012). The financial crisis and the well-being of Americans. *Oxford Economic Papers, 64*(1), 1–26.

Deaton, A. & Stone, A. A. (2016). Understanding context effects for a measure of life evaluation: How responses matter. *Oxford Economic Papers*, 1–10, doi: 10.1093/oep/gpw022

DeJonge, T., Veenhoven, R., Kalmijn, W. M., & Arends, L. R. (2015). Stability of boundaries between response options of response scales. Does 'very happy' remain equally happy over the years? *Social Indicators Research, 123*(1), 241–266. doi:10.1007/s11205-014-0735-2

DeJonge, T., Veenhoven, R., Kalmijn, W. M., & Arends, L. R. (2016). Pooling time series based on slightly different questions about the same topic. Forty years of survey research on happiness and life satisfaction in The Netherlands. *Social Indicators Research, 126*, 863–891. doi:10.1007/s11205-015-0898-5

Dolan, P. & Kavetsos, G. (2012). Happy Talk: Mode of Administration Effects on Subjective Well-Being. *CEP Discussion Paper*, No. 1159. London School of Economics and Political Science. Retrieved May 2014, from http:cep.lse.ac.uk-pubs-download-dp1159.pdf

Howard, G. S., Ralph, K. M., Gulanick, N. A., Maxwell, S. E., Nance, D. W., & Gerber, S. K. (1979). Internal invalidity in pretest-posttest self-report evaluations and a re-evaluation of retrospective pretests, *Applied Psychological Measurement, 3*(1), 1–23. doi:10.1177-014662167900300101

Katz, D. (1942). Do interviewers bias poll results. *The Public Opinion Quarterly, 6*(2), 248–268. Oxford University Press on behalf of the American Association for Public Opinion Research. http:www.jstor.org-stable-2745023.

OECD (2013). OECD guidelines on measuring subjective well-being. OECD Publishing. http:dx.doi.org-10.1787-9789264191655-en

Pudney, S. (2010). An experimental analysis of the impact of survey design on measures and models of subjective wellbeing. *ISER Working Paper Series*, 2010–20. Economic & Social Research Council. Retrieved February 3, 2016, from www.iser.essex.ac.uk/research/publications/working-papers/iser/2010-20.pdf

Schwartz, C. E., & Sudman, S. (Eds.). (1992). *Context effects in social and psychological research.* New York: Springer.

Schwartz, C.E., Ahmed, S., Sawatzky, R., Sajobi, T., Mayo, M., Finkelstein, J., Lix, L., Verdam, M.G.E., Oort, F.J., & Sprangers, M.A.G. (2013). Guidelines for secondary analysis in search of response shift. *Quality of Life Research, 22*, 2663–2673. doi:10.1007-s11136-013-0402-0

Senik, C. (2013). The French Unhappiness Puzzle: the Cultural Dimension of Happiness. Université Paris-Sorbonne and Paris School of Economics. http:www.parisschoolofeconomics.eu-docs-senik-claudia-new_version_french_october25_2013.pdf

Stone, A. A., & Mackie, C. (Eds.). (2013). *Subjective well-being: Measuring happiness, suffering, and other dimensions of experience. Panel on measuring subjective well-being in a policy-relevant framework* . Washington, DC: The National Academies Press.National Research Council, Committee on National Statistics, Division of Behavioral and Social Sciences and Education

Studer, R. & Winkelmann, R. (2014). Reported happiness, fast and slow. *Social Indicators Research, 117*(3), 1055–1067. doi:10.1007-s11205-013-0376-x

van Beuningen, J., van der Houwen, K., & Moonen, L. (2014). Measuring well-being, An analysis of different response scales. Discussion Paper, Statistics Netherlands. Retrieved July 20, 2015, from http:www.cbs.nl-NR-rdonlyres-FF644A99-580C-4D7E-B214-BEE54A947D46-0-Measuringwell being.pdf

Chapter 12
Directions for Further Research

Refinements

Differential Interpretation of Items by Subgroups

In Chap. 4 we described that there are at least two subgroups of the general population that assign an equal value range to equivalent response options for happiness and life satisfaction in The Netherlands. It is possible that other subgroups would evaluate the same response scales differently, but that each subgroup would still evaluate equivalent response options for happiness and life satisfaction in the same way. In addition to this, we found that in Spain at least the subgroup of students does not evaluate equivalent response options for happiness and life satisfaction in the same way. If this difference in evaluation does not hold for the general population, logically there must be at least one other subgroup in each of the two countries that evaluates response options for happiness differently given equivalent options for life satisfaction. In this case this difference in evaluation for this latter subgroup must be different from the evaluation by the students, if it is assumed that a difference in interpretation cannot be found in the general population.

These findings combined with the findings of Chap. 5 that 'very happy' is not always equally happy offer a direction for further research into the differential possible interpretation of response items by subgroups of a general population based on, for example, level of education, type of occupation or age and to compare the outcomes for similar subgroups from different countries. The results of such research will give insight in the extent to which people within subgroups agree on their evaluations of response options and whether this differs between subgroups. It could also shed light on whether a difference or indifference to the interpretation of response options in equivalent scales for different topics is present population wide or just in some subgroups.

T. de Jonge et al., *Diversity in Survey Questions on the Same Topic*, Social Indicators Research Series 68, DOI 10.1007/978-3-319-53261-5_12

Improvement of HSIS Ratings

In the HSIS-studies conducted to date, no attention has been paid to the subjective well-being (SWB) of the judges employed for these studies. Thus we do not know whether the assessment of the boundaries between response options is affected by this SWB. It is desirable to set up a HSIS-study to investigate this, as recommended by Kalmijn (2010, p. 179). In such a study it would also be worthwhile to distinguish between experienced well-being and evaluative well-being of the judges. The first of these two kinds of SWB refers to momentary assessment of affect and the second to appreciation of life as a whole. A person's experienced well-being and evaluative well-being may be very different (Stone and Mackie 2013, pp. 15–16) and thus each of these kinds of SWB may have a different effect on the assessment of the boundaries between response options.

In Chap. 6 we discussed the occurrence of zero-width intervals assigned by judges to anchor points and referred to a more elaborated discussion about this issue in Kalmijn (2010, p. 147 sqq). A suggestion for further research with respect to this matter is to compare the occurrence of such zero-width intervals for the items between groups of native speakers from different countries and to investigate whether there is a cultural pattern in the results. In connection with this, it would be interesting to determine whether there is a relation between the occurrence of zero-width intervals and the '10-excess phenomenon' described in Brulé and Veenhoven (2016) according to which the frequency with which respondents tick a ten stands out and is sometimes higher than the frequency with which a nine is ticked by respondents in the same sample.

The precision of the estimates of the boundaries between response options using the Scale Interval Recorder could be improved, if in future HSIS-studies the number of judges is considerably increased compared to the average number used for studies to date.

The stability over time of the boundaries between response options obtained using the Scale Interval Recorder could be checked by repeating a HSIS-study after an interval of several years using the same or similar subgroups of judges.

Improvement of Estimates Obtained with the Reference Distribution Method

In section "Discussion" of Chap. 11 we mentioned two options for further research on the validation of the Reference Distribution Method. These options were (1) to weigh by the number of respondents to each survey when averaging over the estimated means in a year to pool time series, (2) to repeat the process of pooling time series with the other waves of the World Values Survey (WVS) that are available for this, to obtain a more stable pooled time series that is less prone to systematic errors.

The main emphasis of this book has been placed on the introduction of new techniques to deal with the comparability problem caused by differences in survey items used the measure the same latent variable. We have restricted the inspection of time series to distortions caused by the influential factors discussed in section "Distortion of trends due to biases in measurement", and especially the influence of changes in the mode of surveying. Although we pooled time series from different surveys, we have not paid attention to the quality of the data sources used in terms as for instance the non-response, the selectivity of the response, and whether or not correction methods such as re-weighting of the results have been applied. To improve the reliability of the pooled time series, it is necessary to investigate the quality of the data sources and to decide which data sources meet the required quality and which data sources do not.

In addition to the preceding points, it would be interesting to repeat the process of pooling time series by deriving initial reference distributions from survey results measured using other numerical scales than those taken from the WVS to investigate whether this would lead to similar outcomes. Candidate response scales for such an exercise are, for example, the 10-point scales of the items life satisfaction from the European Social Survey and European Quality of Life Survey.

From the perspective of international comparisons, it is sensible to investigate how much difference it makes whether a 10-point or an 11-point numerical scale is used to derive a reference distribution from. In both cases, the primary numerical scale has to be transformed to fit into the 0–10 continuum. For a 10-point scale this corresponds to shifting down the ranks of all the response options by 0.5 (Kalmijn 2013). The differences in sample means between countries when based on the Weighted Average Approach would therefore not change due to the transformation of the 10-point scale. If an 11-point numerical scale is used, however, the value of the response options with a rank lower than 5 would be higher on the transformed scale than the rank on the primary scale, whereas the value of the other response options ranked higher than 5 would be lower than the rank of the primary scale. The transformation of the 11-point numerical scale would thus affect the differences between the samples means according to the Weighted Average Approach. There is a need to investigate whether this difference in effect of using a 10-point or 11-point scale as a basis for the Reference Distribution Method is of importance for the conclusions that can be drawn from the results of the application of this method.

The 10-excess phenomenon which we referred to in section "Improvement of HSIS ratings" does not occur as often within a country Brulé and Veenhoven (2016). This asks for research to find out what the impact of the 10-excess phenomenon is on the derivation of a reference distribution and what solutions can be found to assure that this impact does not come at the cost of the validity of an international comparison.

Comparison of the Estimates Obtained with the HSIS and the Reference Distribution Method

In section "Comparison of the estimated means using different methods" we have demonstrated that the combination of the assessment of boundaries between response options using the Happiness Scale Interval Recorder and the Continuum Approach cannot be used to solve the comparability problem. We explained that this may be due to the fact that a verbal response scale does not necessarily offer response options that meet the perception of respondents well, which may force them to choose between two less than optimal alternatives. As a consequence, the boundaries between response options obtained using the Scale Interval Method differ dramatically from the boundaries derived from a reference distribution as done in the Reference Distribution Method, which we illustrated in Fig. 8.2 of section "Illustration of applying the reference distribution method". From a scientific point of view, it would be of interest to study how the boundaries found using the Scale Interval Method differ from boundaries obtained using the Reference Distribution Method for a number of countries from all over the world to find out whether groups of countries can be detected for which these differences are similar and whether this can be attributed to cultural differences. The results of such a study would contribute to increasing our insight into the extent to which language and culture affect the interpretation of response options in surveys and, as a corollary, the response of individual respondents to survey questions.

Applications

Application in Research Synthesis of Happiness

The innovations we have presented in this book were all developed in the context of the World Database of Happiness (WDH), the main aim of which is to gather the available research findings on happiness and prepare these data for research synthesis. We will discuss some of the options for synthetic analysis in this section.

Distributional findings on happiness based on survey questions that validly tap an individual's 'overall appreciation of life as a whole' are presented in the WDH collection of these findings. These distributional findings include a mean and standard deviation, and comparison of data within and across countries is facilitated by a transformation to a 0–10 scale. The current transformations are based on the traditional methods described in sections "Linear stretch" and "Semantic judgment of fixed word value". A better alternative is to apply the Reference Distribution Method. Reference distributions are now available for several items for almost all countries in the world, for instance the 0–10 life satisfaction items used in Gallup World Poll and the European Social Survey.

The pooling of time series discussed in Chap. 11 allows presenting longer time series for happiness and life satisfaction in the WDH and allows us to study trends in these topics over a longer time span than is possible at this moment. In section "Discussion" we have stated that the estimated population mean of a reference distribution can serve as a reference value for comparison purposes, but it should not be considered to be the 'true' value of the perception of happiness or life satisfaction on the continuum from 0 to 10. Other reference distributions may constitute a different reference value. If we assume, however, that a reference value is mainly determinant for bringing survey results to a comparable level, but does not affect the pattern of the trend of a time series, than the trends of different pooled time series which are based on different reference distributions can be compared.

A thorough analysis of the results from all the HSIS-studies that have been conducted would be helpful to detect groups of countries where response scales are interpreted similarly and to identify for which response scale this is the case. A comparison of the level of happiness between countries within those groups will be more reliable since no differential interpretation of the response scales has to be taken into account.

Application in New Research on Happiness

From the comparison of the assessments by judges from different countries, described in Chaps. 4, 5, and 6, it is clear that results for one country cannot be generalized to other languages and cultures. An extended study using the Scale Interval Recorder would contribute to investigating further the hypothesis of Saris and Andreenkova (2001), that the relationship between happiness and satisfaction with life varies with the cultural and linguistic environment in which it is studied.

People in different countries may speak the same language, but, due to cultural influences, they may not interpret response scales in the same way. The Scale Interval Recorder offers an opportunity to study the differences in interpretation of response options by native speakers of one language, living in different countries or from different subcultures. Examples of languages and countries would be Chinese and China, Malaysia and other countries where Chinese is a primary language for a cultural group, French and France, Canada, Belgium, Morocco, Haiti and Switzerland where French is a primary language for cultural groups, or English and Great Britain, the United States, Canada, New Zealand and South Africa where English is a primary language for cultural groups.

A variant on the study described above, would be to compare the interpretation of response options by groups of native speakers who live in the same country but speak a different language, such as in Switzerland or Belgium. The aim of this type of research comes close to the research reported in a paper by Senik (2013), who compares the happiness of French natives with the happiness of immigrants living inside and outside France and to that of the survey study by Van der Houwen and

Moonen (2014), who compare the happiness of Dutch natives with that of immigrants.

If such cultural differences in response to identical items appear to exist, the next step is to correct for this. This involves the computation of adjusted means and standard deviations and subsequent assessment of the predictive validity of these.

Application to Other Topics Than Happiness

In section "Implication of the method" we introduced the term 'translation bias' for the phenomenon that an adverb used in the label of a response options is not necessarily always translated by using the same adverb in another language, such as when the translation in Spanish of the adverb 'Fairly' in the label 'Fairly satisfied' in English would be 'Más bien' for one scale and 'Bastante' for another scale. To improve the comparison of happiness across nations it is of importance to gain more uniformity in the translation of adverbs. Therefore it is necessary to get more insight in the size of the translation bias in terms of the frequency of occurrence in different countries. To reduce the diversity in adverbs used in a language for the translation of a single adverb in another language, the Happiness Scale Interval Recorder can be used as an instrument to get insight into the extent to which different adverbs are interpreted differently in the context of the scale and the keyword of concern. We recommend not to restrict this to the keywords happiness and satisfaction, but to include response options labeled with other keywords. In European socio-economic and opinion surveys which are mentioned on the website[1] of the European Data Center for Work and Welfare (EDAC), we found, for example, response options labeled with the adverb 'fairly' in combination with a number of keywords such as 'easily', 'difficult', 'likely', 'safe', 'good' and 'bad'.

In this book we have considered the comparability problem only from the perspective of happiness and, to a limited extent, satisfaction with the way democracy in the country one lives in works. The comparability problem, however, is ubiquitous throughout social science research for a range of topics, such as how satisfied people are with their housing, working conditions or their present job, but also how safe they feel when walking alone in their neighborhood at night, how they assess their own health, how interested they are in politics or how well they are able to make ends meet given their household income. Examples of the survey items and the diversity of response scales used can be found in the surveys mentioned at the previously introduced website of EDAC and also in surveys of National Statistical Offices. Besides social science research there are also other fields of research which have to cope with the comparability problem. Two fields of research in which the comparability problem is as prominent as it is in happiness research are those of consumer satisfaction (Bartikowski et al. 2010) and of

[1]http://www.edac.eu/

customer satisfaction (MORI 2002; Braunsberger and Gates 2009; Danaher and Haddrell 1996). What makes customer satisfaction especially interesting from the perspective of the interpretation of response items is that it is of concern to parties in both the private and public sector. With respect to the comparability problem the field of health research is also worth mentioning, here the perceptions people have of their physical functioning, of the pain they experience or of their mental well-being are measured (Schwartz and Sprangers 1999; McDowell 2006; Davis et al. 2010). As in happiness research and the other fields of research we referred to, the differences in response scales and language used over time and between countries and subgroups of the population makes comparison of survey results in health research difficult.

Based on the preceding we recommend making an inventory of other topics within the social sciences and other fields of science, for which the perceptions of people have been measured using survey research and discrete scales over a long period of time, and for which the comparability problem is a serious issue. Based on this inventory and the results of, and directions given for further research in this book, a plan can be made for research to address the comparability problem found in these fields. This would also give us an opportunity to determine whether or not using the family of beta distributions is appropriate for other topics than happiness and life satisfaction to convert time series and, if so, or not, to determine and further develop the methods that are most appropriate to use in these situations.

References

Bartikowski, B., Kamei, K., & Chandon, J. L. (2010). A verbal rating scale to measure Japanese consumers' perceptions of product quality. *Asia Pacific Journal of Marketing and Logistics, 22* (2), 179–195. doi:10.1108/13555851011026935

Braunsberger, B., & Gates, R. (2009). Developing inventories for satisfaction and Likert scales in a service environment. *Journal of Services Marketing, 23*(4), 219–225. doi 10.1108/08876040910965557

Brulé, G., & Veenhoven, V. (2016). The '10-excess' phenomenon in responses to survey questions on happiness. *Social Indicators Research*, Published online: 30 March 2016. doi:10.1007/s11205–016-1265-x

Danaher, P. J., & Haddrell, V. (1996). A comparison of question scales used for measuring customer satisfaction. *International Journal of Service Industry Management, 7*(4), 4–26.

Davis, R. E., Couper, M. P., Janz, N. K., Caldwell, C. H., & Resnicow, K. (2010). Interviewer effects in public health surveys. *Health Education Research, 25*(1), 14–26. Oxford University Press, doi 10.1093-her-cyp046.

Houwen, K van der., & Moonen, L. (2014). Allochtonen en geluk. Bevolkingstrends 2014(10), Statistics Netherlands

Kalmijn, W. M. (2010). Quantification of happiness inequality. Dissertation, Erasmus University Rotterdam, The Netherlands. Enschede: Ipskamp Drukkers. Available at http://repub.eur.nl/pub/21777

Kalmijn, W. M. (2013). From discrete 1 to 10 towards continuous 0 to 10: The continuum approach to estimating the distribution of happiness in a nation. *Social Indicators Research, 110*(2), 549–557. doi 10.1007-s11205-011-9943-1

McDowell, I. (2006). *Measuring health. A guide to rating scales and questionnaires* (3rd ed.). Oxford: Oxford University Press. http://a4ebm.org/sites/default/files/Measuring%20Health.pdf.

MORI (2002). *Public service reform. Measuring and understanding customer satisfaction*. London: MORI Social Research Institute. Retrieved January 29, 2016, from https://www.ipsos-mori.com/DownloadPublication/1202_sri_local_gov_public-service_reform_measuring_and_understanding_customer_satisfaction_042002.PDF

Saris, W. E., & Andreenkova, A. (2001). Following changes in living conditions and happiness in post communist Russia: The Russet panel. *Journal of Happiness Studies, 2*, 95–109. doi:10.1023/A:1011579608121

Schwartz, C. E., & Sprangers, M. A. G. (1999). Methodological approaches for assessing response shift in longitudinal health-related quality-of-life research. *Social Science & Medicine, 48*, 1531–1548.

Senik, C. (2013). The French unhappiness puzzle: The cultural dimension of happiness. Université Paris-Sorbonne and Paris School of Economics. http:www.parisschoolofeconomics.eu-docs-senik-claudia-new_version_french_october25_2013.pdf

Stone, A. A., & Mackie, C. (Eds.). (2013). *Subjective well-being: Measuring happiness, suffering, and other dimensions of experience. Panel on measuring subjective well-being in a policy-relevant framework*. Washington, DC: National Research Council, Committee on National Statistics, Division of Behavioral and Social Sciences and Education, The National Academies Press.

Appendices

Appendix A: Original and English Wording of Survey Items on Happiness from the Non-English HSIS-Studies Used in This Book (Tables A.1 and A.2)

For an explanation of the question codes in the last column, see Table 1.1 in Chap. 1.

Table A.1 Items from the Dutch HSIS-studies

Wording in Dutch	Wording in English	Question code
Voelde u zich de afgelopen 4 weken gelukkig?	During the last 4 weeks, did you feel happy?	M-FH-cm-sq-v-5-b
Voortdurend	All of the time	
Meestal	Most of the time	
Soms	Some of the time	
Zelden	Seldom	
Nooit	Never	
Voelt u zich	Do you feel……?	M-FH-u-sq-v-3-a
Gelukkig	Happy	
Niet zo gelukkig	Not very happy	
Ongelukkig	Unhappy	
Hoe tevreden bent u met uw leven in het algemeen?	How satisfied are you with your life in general?	O-SLu-g-sq-v-5-c
Volledig tevreden	Completely satisfied	
Tevreden	Satisfied	
Niet tevreden, niet ontevreden	Unsatisfied nor satisfied	
Ontevreden	Unsatisfied	
Volledig ontevreden	Completely unsatisfied	

(continued)

T. de Jonge et al., *Diversity in Survey Questions on the Same Topic*, Social Indicators Research Series 68, DOI 10.1007/978-3-319-53261-5

Table A.1 (continued)

Wording in Dutch	Wording in English	Question code
Vindt u zichzelf gelukkig?	Are you happy with your life?	O-HL-u-sq-v-2-a
Ja	Yes	
Nee	No	
In welke mate vindt u zichzelf een gelukkig mens?	To what extent do you consider yourself a happy person....?	O-HP-u-sq-v-5-d (pair 2, section "Response options labeled in Dutch")
Erg gelukkig	Very happy	
Gelukkig	Happy	
Niet gelukkig, niet ongelukkig	Neither happy nor unhappy	
Ongelukkig	Unhappy	
Erg ongelukkig	Very unhappy	
In welke mate bent u tevreden met het leven dat u op dit moment leidt?	To what extent are you satisfied with the life you currently lead?	O-SLL-c-sq-v-5-d (pair 3, section "Response options labeled in Dutch")
Buitengewoon tevreden	Extraordinarily satisfied	
Zeer tevreden	Very satisfied	
Tevreden	Satisfied	
Tamelijk tevreden	Fairly satisfied	
Niet zo tevreden	Not very satisfied	
Ik ben erg gelukkig met het leven dat ik leid	I am very happy with the kind of life I lead	O-SLL-u-sq-v-5a
Helemaal mee eens	Strongly agree	
Mee eens	Agree	
Niet mee eens, niet mee oneens	Neither agree nor disagree	
Niet mee eens	Disagree	
Helemaal niet mee eens	Strongly disagree	
In welke mate bent u tevreden met het leven dat u op dit moment leidt?	To what extent are you satisfied with the life you currently lead?	O-SLL-c-sq-v-5-f (pair 2, section "Response options labeled in Dutch")
Erg tevreden	Very satisfied	
Tevreden	Satisfied	
Niet tevreden, niet ontevreden	Neither satisfied, nor dissatisfied	
Ontevreden	Dissatisfied	
Erg ontevreden	Very dissatisfied	
In welke mate vindt u zichzelf een gelukkig mens?	To what extent do you consider yourself a happy person....?	O-HP-u-sq-v-5-a (pair 3, section "Response options labeled in Dutch")
Erg gelukkig	Very happy	
Gelukkig	Happy	
Niet gelukkig, niet ongelukkig	Neither happy nor unhappy	
Niet zo gelukkig	Not very happy	
Ongelukkig	Unhappy	

(continued)

Table A.1 (continued)

Wording in Dutch	Wording in English	Question code
Nu een vraag over de manier waarop u op het ogenblik vooruit komt: bent u daarover	How satisfied are you with the way you are getting on now?	O-SLS-c-sq-v-3-ab
Zeer tevreden	Very satisfied	
Tevreden	Satisfied	
Ontevreden	Not satisfied	
Vindt u zichzelf......?	Do you think of yourself as.......?	O-HP-u-sq-v-3-a
Gelukkig	Happy	
Tamelijk gelukkig	Fairly happy	
Ongelukkig	Unhappy	
Hoe gelukkig bent u, alles bijeengenomen?	Taking all things together, would you say you are.....?	O-HL-u-sq-v-4-a (pair 1, section "Response options labeled in Dutch")
Heel gelukkig	Very happy	
Tamelijk gelukkig	Fairly happy	
Niet zo gelukkig	Not very happy	
Helemaal niet gelukkig	Not at all happy	
Hoe gelukkig of ongelukkig bent u met uw leven in het algemeen?	If you were to consider your life in general, how happy or unhappy would you say you are, on the whole?	O-HL-g-sq-v-7-a
Volkomen gelukkig	Completely happy	
Zeer gelukkig	Very happy	
Tamelijk gelukkig	Fairly happy	
Noch gelukkig, noch ongelukkig	Neither happy nor unhappy	
Tamelijk ongelukkig	Fairly unhappy	
Zeer ongelukkig	Very unhappy	
Volkomen ongelukkig	Completely unhappy	
Hoe tevreden bent u over het algemeen met het leven dat u leidt?	On the whole how satisfied are you with the life you lead?	O-SLL-u-sq-v-4-b (pair 1, section "Response options labeled in Dutch")
Zeer tevreden	Very satisfied	
Tamelijk tevreden	Fairly satisfied	
Niet zo tevreden	Not very satisfied	
Helemaal niet tevreden	Not at all satisfied	
Hoe tevreden bent u met uw leven in het algemeen op dit moment?	How satisfied are you with your life in general these days?	O-SLW-c-sq-v-5-fb
Zeer tevreden	Very satisfied	
Tamelijk tevreden	Fairly satisfied	
Tevreden noch ontevreden	Satisfied nor dissatisfied	
Tamelijk ontevreden	Fairly dissatisfied	
Zeer ontevreden	Very dissatisfied	

(continued)

Table A.1 (continued)

Wording in Dutch	Wording in English	Question code
In welke mate vindt u zichzelf een gelukkig mens?	To what extent do you consider yourself a happy person....?	O-HP-u-sq-v-5-h
Buitengewoon gelukkig	Extraordinarily happy	
Zeer gelukkig	Very happy	
Gelukkig	Happy	
Tamelijk gelukkig	Fairly happy	
Niet zo gelukkig	Not very happy	
Over het algemeen kan ik zeggen dat ik min of meer het leven leidt dat ik wil leiden	On the whole my life is close to how I would like it to be	C-RA-u-sq-v-5-a
Volledig akkoord	Strongly agree	
Akkoord	Agree	
Noch akkoord, noch niet akkoord	Neither agree nor disagree	
Niet akkoord	Disagree	
Helemaal niet akkoord	Strongly disagree	
Voelt u zichzelf.	Do you feel. . . . . ..?	M-FH-u-sq-v-3-d
Gelukkig	Happy	
Tamelijk gelukkig	Fairly happy	
Ongelukkig	Unhappy	
Hoe vaak gedurende de afgelopen 4 weken was u een gelukkig mens?	During the past 4 weeks. . ... Have you been a happy person?	M-TH-cm-sq-v-6-a
Altijd	All of the time	
Meestal	Most of the time	
Vaak	A good bit of the time	
Soms	Some of the time	
Zelden	A little of the time	
Nooit	None of the time	
Voelde u zich de afgelopen 4 weken gelukkig?	During the last 4 weeks, did you feel happy?	M-TH-cm-sq-v-5-c
Voortdurend	Always	
Vaak	Often	
Soms	Sometimes	
Zelden	Seldom	
Nooit	Never	

Table A.2 Items from the Spanish HSIS-study

Wording in Spanish	Wording in English	Question code
En general, ¿diría Ud. que está . . . con el tipo de vida que lleva?	On the whole how satisfied are you with the life you lead	O-SLL-u-sq-v-4-b
Muy satisfecho/a	Very satisfied	
Más bien satisfecho/a	Fairly satisfied	
No muy satisfecho/a	Not very satisfied	
Nada satisfecho/a	Not at all satisfied	
En general, tal y como están las cosas hoy en día, ¿cómo diría usted que es hoy en día?	Taken all together, how would you say things are these days? Would you say that you are....?	O-HL-c-sq-v-3-ab (pair 1, section "Response options labeled in Spanish")
Muy feliz	Very happy	
Bastante feliz	Fairly happy	
No muy feliz	Not too happy	
En general, tal y como están las cosas hoy en día, ¿cómo diría usted que es hoy en día?	Taken all together, how would you say things are these days? Would you say you are:	O-HL-c-sq-v-4-g
Muy feliz	Very happy	
Bastante feliz	Pretty happy	
No muy feliz	Not too happy	
Muy infeliz	Very unhappy	
En términos generales, ¿diría Ud. que está satisfecho/a con su vida? Diría Ud. que está . . .	In general, would you say that you are satisfied with your life?	O-Slu-g-sq-v-4-c (pair 2, section "Response options labeled in Spanish")
Muy satisfecho/a	Very satisfied	
Bastante satisfecho/a	Fairly satisfied	
No muy satisfecho/a	Not very satisfied	
Para nada satisfecho/a	Not at all satisfied	
En términos generales, diría Ud. que está satisfecho/a con su vida? Diría Ud. que está.	In general, would you say that you are satisfied with your life? Would you say that you are . . .	O-SLu-g-sq-v-4-b
Muy satisfecho/a	Very satisfied	
Bastante satisfecho/a	Quite satisfied	
Satisfecho/a	Satisfied	
No muy satisfecho/a	Not very satisfied	
En líneas generales, ¿diría Ud. que es. . .?	Taking all things together, would you say you are.....?	O-HL-u-sq-v-4-a (pair 2, section "Response options labeled in Spanish")
Muy feliz	Very happy	
Bastante feliz	Quite happy	
No muy feliz	Not very happy	
Nada feliz	Not at all happy	
En general, teniendo todo en cuenta, ¿cómo ve Ud. su situación actual? Diría que actualmente es Ud. . . .	Taking all things together, how would you say things are these days? Would you say you are..?	O-HL-c-sq-v-4-g
Muy feliz	Very happy	
Bastante feliz	Pretty happy	
Poco feliz	Not too happy	
Nada feliz	Very unhappy	

(continued)

Table A.2 (continued)

Wording in Spanish	Wording in English	Question code
¿Como satisfecho/a está usted con cómo le está yendo actualmente?	In general, would you say that you are satisfied with your life?	O-SLS-C-sq-v-3-ab (pair 1, section "Response options labeled in Spanish")
Muy satisfecho/a	Very satisfied	
Bastante satisfecho/a	Fairly satisfied	
No muy satisfecho/a	Not very satisfied	
Teniendo en cuenta su vida en general, ¿cómo se considera Ud.?	If you were to consider your life in general, how happy of unhappy would you say you are, on the whole?	O-HL-g-sq-v-7-a
Completamente feliz	Completely happy	
Muy feliz	Very happy	
Bastante feliz	Fairly happy	
Ni feliz, ni desdichado/a	Neither happy nor unhappy	
Bastante desdichado/a	Fairly unhappy	
Muy desdichado/a	Very unhappy	
Completamente desdichado/a	Completely unhappy	
Por lo general, ¿está usted satisfecho con su vida? Señale el número que mejor describa cómo se siente	Taken all things together, how satisfied are you with your life as a whole these days? On the whole, would you say you are.....?	O-SLW-c-sq-v-5-g
Muy satisfecho/a	Very satisfied	
Satisfecho/a	Satisfied	
Neutro/a	Neither satisfied nor dissatisfied	
Insatisfecho/a	Dissatisfied	
Muy insatisfecho/a	Very dissatisfied	

Appendix B: Statistics of the Assessments by Students in the HSIS-Studies Used (Tables B.1, B.2, B.3, B.4, B.5, B.6, and B.7)

In this appendix we report the main statistics of the assessments by students of the items in the HSIS-studies used in this book. The total number of participating students for each study is given in the header of the table. Only the number of valid assessments is given for each item. An assessment is invalid if, for example, a judge has placed all the sliders of the Scale Interval Recorder in the same position on the scale. Rules for skipping these invalid assessments are given by Kalmijn (2010, pp. 144–145).

Table B.1 Assessments by 204 Dutch students of items from Dutch6

Item	Question code (valid assessments)	Upper boundary	Standard deviation	Standard error	# zero-width
During the last 4 weeks, did you feel happy?					
All of the time	M-FH-cm-sq-v-5-b (195)	10.0			12
Most of the time		8.5	0.73	0.05	
Some of the time		5.9	1.07	0.08	
Seldom		3.6	1.15	0.08	37
Never		1.3	1.00	0.07	
Do you feel. . .. . ..?					
Happy	M-FH-u-sq-v-3-a (195)	10.0			1
Not very happy		6.4	1.40	0.10	
Unhappy		3.1	1.34	0.10	8
How satisfied are you with your life in general?					
Completely satisfied	O-SLu-g-sq-v-5-c (194)	10.0			
Satisfied		8.5	0.78	0.32	13
Unsatisfied nor satisfied		5.9	1.01	0.42	
Unsatisfied		4.0	1.19	0.49	
Completely unsatisfied		1.5	1.12	0.46	29
Are you happy with your life?					
Yes	O-HL-u-sq-v-2-a (192)	10.0			-
No		5.8	1.43	0.10	
To what extent do you consider yourself a happy person....?					
Very happy	O-HP-u-sq-v-5-d (194)	10.0			3
Happy		8.3	0.76	0.05	
Neither happy nor unhappy		5.8	1.15	0.08	
Unhappy		4.0	1.27	0.09	
Very unhappy		1.6	1.01	0.07	18
To what extent are you satisfied with the life you currently lead?					
Extraordinarily satisfied	O-SLL-c-sq-v-5-d (196)	10.0			15
Very satisfied		8.9	0.70	0.05	
Satisfied		7.1	1.02	0.07	
Fairly satisfied		5.2	1.46	0.10	
Not very satisfied		3.5	1.83	0.13	10
I am very happy with the kind of life I lead					
Strongly agree	O-SLL-u-sq-v-5a (192)	10.0			13
Agree		8.6	0.72	0.05	
Neither agree nor disagree		6.0	1.02	0.07	
Disagree		4.1	1.20	0.09	
Strongly disagree		1.7	1.18	0.09	22

(continued)

Table B.1 (continued)

Item	Question code (valid assessments)	Upper boundary	Standard deviation	Standard error	# zero-width
To what extent are you satisfied with the life you currently lead?					
Very satisfied	O-SLL-c-sq-v-5-f (193)	10.0			5
Satisfied		8.4	0.77	0.06	
Neither satisfied, nor dissatisfied		5.8	1.04	0.07	
Dissatisfied		4.0	1.18	0.08	
Very dissatisfied		1.8	1.09	0.08	15
To what extent do you consider yourself a happy person....?					
Very happy	O-HP-u-sq-v-5-a (191)	10.0			4
Happy		8.5	0.67	0.05	
Neither happy nor unhappy		5.9	1.08	0.08	
Not very happy		4.1	1.28	0.09	
Unhappy		2.1	1.34	0.10	19
How satisfied are you with the way you are getting on now?					
Very satisfied	O-SLS-c-sq-v-3-ab (196)	10.0			3
Satisfied		7.9	0.87	0.06	
Not satisfied		4.3	1.65	0.12	3

Table B.2 Assessments by 184 Dutch students of items from Dutch7

Item	Question code (valid assessments)	Upper boundary	Standard deviation	Standard error	# zero-width
Do you think of yourself as.......?					
Happy	O-HP-u-sq-v-3-a (181)	10.0			1
Fairly happy		7.2	0.96	0.07	
Unhappy		4.2	1.55	0.11	2
Taking all things together, would you say you are.....?					
Very happy	O-HL-u-sq-v-4-a (176)	10.0			6
Fairly happy		7.9	0.99	0.07	
Not very happy		5.1	1.26	0.09	
Not at all happy		2.9	1.49	0.11	12
If you were to consider your life in general, how happy or unhappy would you say you are, on the whole?					
Completely happy	O-HL-g-sq-v-7-a (158)	10.0			33
Very happy		9.2	0.72	0.06	
Fairly happy		7.5	0.79	0.06	
Neither happy nor unhappy		5.6	0.75	0.06	
Fairly unhappy		4.3	0.81	0.06	
Very unhappy		2.8	0.89	0.07	
Completely unhappy		1.1	0.85	0.07	35

(continued)

Table B.2 (continued)

Item	Question code (valid assessments)	Upper boundary	Standard deviation	Standard error	# zero-width
On the whole how satisfied are you with the life you lead?					
Very satisfied	O-SLL-u-sq-v-4-b (176)	10.0			5
Fairly satisfied		7.8	0.84	0.06	
Not very satisfied		5.1	1.23	0.09	
Not at all satisfied		2.9	1.51	0.11	14
How satisfied are you with your life in general these days?					
Very satisfied	O-SLW-c-sq-v-5-fb (171)	10.0			5
Fairly satisfied		8.1	0.79	0.06	
Satisfied nor dissatisfied		5.7	0.93	0.07	
Fairly dissatisfied		4.2	1.09	0.08	
Very dissatisfied		2.3	1.27	0.10	15
To what extent do you consider yourself a happy person....?					
Extraordinarily happy	O-HP-u-sq-v-5-h (172)	10.0			19
Very happy		8.9	0.75	0.06	
Happy		7.3	0.89	0.07	
Fairly happy		5.5	1.42	0.11	
Not very happy		3.7	1.82	0.14	11
On the whole my life is close to how I would like it to be					
Strongly agree	C-RA-u-sq-v-5-a (164)	10.0			28
Agree		8.7	1.02	0.08	
Neither agree nor disagree		5.9	0.93	0.07	
Disagree		4.3	1.12	0.09	
Strongly disagree		2.0	1.33	0.10	18
Do you feel.......?					
Happy	M-FH-u-sq-v-3-d (179)	10.0			1
Fairly happy		7.1	1.17	0.09	
Unhappy		4.0	1.66	0.12	9
During the past 4 weeks..... Have you been a happy person?					
All of the time	M-TH-cm-sq-v-6-a (160)	10.0			33
Most of the time		9.1	0.66	0.05	
A good bit of the time		7.2	0.87	0.07	
Some of the time		5.5	1.12	0.09	
A little of the time		3.6	1.30	0.10	
None of the time		1.4	1.28	0.10	35

(continued)

Table B.2 (continued)

Item	Question code (valid assessments)	Upper boundary	Standard deviation	Standard error	# zero-width
During the last 4 weeks. Did you feel happy?					
Always	M-TH-cm-sq-v-5-c (165)	10.0			20
Often		8.7	0.94	0.07	
Sometimes		6.2	1.03	0.08	
Seldom		4.0	1.26	0.10	
Never		1.8	1.35	0.11	27

Table B.3 Assessments by 427 Spanish students of items from Spanish9

Item	Question code (valid assessments)	Upper boundary	Standard deviation	Standard error	# zero-width
On the whole how satisfied are you with the life you lead					
Very satisfied	O-SLL-u-sq-v-4-b (391)	10.0			52
Fairly satisfied		8.4	1.33	0.07	
Not very satisfied		5.5	1.43	0.07	
Not at all satisfied		2.5	1.70	0.09	33
Taken all together, how would you say things are these days? Would you say that you are....?					
Very happy	O-HL-c-sq-v-3-ab (400)	10.0			30
Fairly happy		7.7	1.57	0.08	
Not too happy		3.4	1.92	0.10	23
Taken all together, how would you say things are these days? Would you say you are:					
Very happy	O-HL-c-sq-v-4-g (378)	10.0			37
Pretty happy		8.2	1.29	0.07	
Not too happy		4.6	1.60	0.08	
Very unhappy		1.7	1.45	0.07	62
In general, would you say that you are satisfied with your life?					
Very satisfied	O-Slu-g-sq-v-4-c (371)	10.0			39
Fairly satisfied		8.2	1.34	0.07	
Not very satisfied		4.6	1.74	0.09	
Not at all satisfied		1.6	1.49	0.08	72
In general, would you say that you are satisfied with your life? Would you say that you are . . .					
Very satisfied	O-SLu-g-sq-v-4-b (395)	10.0			42
Quite satisfied		8.3	1.40	0.07	
Satisfied		5.5	1.66	0.08	
Not very satisfied		2.5	1.83	0.09	55
Taking all things together, would you say you are.....?					
Very happy	O-HL-u-sq-v-4-a (389)	10.0			92
Quite happy		8.8	1.20	0.06	
Not very happy		6.1	1.69	0.09	
Not at all happy		3.0	2.06	0.10	64

(continued)

Table B.3 (continued)

Item	Question code (valid assessments)	Upper boundary	Standard deviation	Standard error	# zero-width
Taking all things together, how would you say things are these days? Would you say you are..?					
Very happy	O-HL-c-sq-v-4-g (369)	10.0			40
Pretty happy		8.2	1.33	0.07	
Not too happy		4.6	1.69	0.09	
Very unhappy		1.6	1.64	0.09	86
In general, would you say that you are satisfied with your life?					
Very satisfied	O-SLS-C-sq-v-3-ab (388)	10.0			28
Fairly satisfied		7.7	1.53	0.08	
Not very satisfied		3.3	2.05	0.10	29
If you were to consider your life in general, how happy of unhappy would you say you are, on the whole?					
Completely happy	O-HL-g-sq-v-7-a (300)	10.0			96
Very happy		9.3	0.80	0.05	
Fairly happy		7.4	0.93	0.05	
Neither happy nor unhappy		5.3	1.01	0.06	
Fairly unhappy		3.6	0.93	0.05	
Very unhappy		2.0	0.82	0.05	
Completely unhappy		0.6	0.80	0.05	138
Taken all things together. How satisfied are you with your life as a whole these days? On the whole would you say you are.....?					
Very satisfied	O-SLW-c-sq-v-5-g (325)	10.0			39
Satisfied		8.5	1.12	0.06	
Neither satisfied nor dissatisfied		5.5	1.29	0.07	
Dissatisfied		3.4	1.27	0.07	
Very dissatisfied		1.1	1.11	0.06	90

Table B.4 Assessments by 348 American students of items from English9

Item	Question code (valid assessments)	Upper boundary	Standard deviation	Standard error	# zero-width
In general, how happy would you say you are?					
Very happy	O-HL-g-sq-v-3-a (340)	10.0			12
Fairly happy		7.6	1.23	0.07	
Not at all happy		3.4	1.59	0.09	6
Taken all together, how would you say things are these days? Would you say that you are....?					
Very happy	O-HL-c-sq-v-3-aa (335) (*item intended was* O-HL-g-sq-v-3-j)	10.0			9
Pretty happy		7.6	1.22	0.07	
Not too happy		3.5	1.64	0.09	10
If you were to consider your life in general these days, how happy or unhappy would you say you are, on the whole...?					
Very happy	O-HL-c-sq-v-4-f (326)	10.0			11
Fairly happy		7.9	1.07	0.06	
Not very happy		4.3	1.38	0.08	
Not at all happy		1.7	1.32	0.07	34
If you were to consider your life in general, how happy or unhappy would you say you are on the whole?					
Very happy	O-HL-u-sq-v-4-g (325) (*item intended was* O-HL-u-sq-v-4-a)	10.0			16
Fairly happy		7.9	1.18	0.07	
Fairly unhappy		4.3	1.32	0.07	
Very unhappy		1.7	1.19	0.07	33
Presently, would you describe yourself as					
Very happy	O-HL-g-sq-v-4-b (323)	10.0			13
Somewhat happy		7.8	1.18	0.07	
Somewhat unhappy		4.4	1.42	0.08	
Very unhappy		1.6	1.26	0.07	19
Taking all things together, would you say you are.....?					
Very happy	O-HL-u-sq-v-4-ac (321)	10.0			13
Rather happy		7.9	1.08	0.06	
Not very happy		4.4	1.31	0.07	
Not at all happy		1.7	1.21	0.07	29

(continued)

Table B.4 (continued)

Item	Question code (valid assessments)	Upper boundary	Standard deviation	Standard error	# zero-width
How happy do you feel as you live now? Please choose one item on this card that comes closest to your feeling					
Very happy	O-HL-c-sq-v-5-e (313)	10.0			15
Fairly happy		8.1	0.94	0.05	
Neither happy nor unhappy		5.4	1.08	0.06	
Fairly unhappy		3.5	1.12	0.06	
Very unhappy		1.4	0.96	0.05	29
Taking all things together in your life, how would you say things are these days? Would you say you are....?					
Very happy	O-HL-c-sq-v-5-a (310)	10.0			9
Happy		8.2	0.83	0.05	
Neither happy nor unhappy		5.5	0.97	0.06	
Unhappy		3.6	1.00	0.06	
Very unhappy		1.4	0.86	0.05	30
If you were to consider your life in general, how happy or unhappy would you say you are, on the whole?					
Completely happy	O-HL-g-sq-v-7-a (295)	10.0			90
Very happy		9.3	0.73	0.04	
Fairly happy		7.3	0.87	0.05	
Neither happy nor unhappy		5.3	0.78	0.05	
Fairly unhappy		3.8	0.79	0.05	
Very unhappy		2.1	0.77	0.04	
Completely unhappy		0.5	0.64	0.04	117
During the past 4 weeks. . ... Have you been a happy person?					

(continued)

Table B.4 (continued)

Item	Question code (valid assessments)	Upper boundary	Standard deviation	Standard error	# zero-width
All of the time	M-TH-cm-sq-v-6-a (292)	10.0			96
Most of the time		9.2	0.91	0.05	
A good bit of the time		6.9	1.08	0.06	
Some of the time		4.7	1.16	0.07	
A little of the time		2.7	1.05	0.06	
None of the time		0.6	0.92	0.05	133

Table B.5 Assessments by 270 American students of items from English10

Item	Question code (valid assessments)	Upper boundary	Standard deviation	Standard error	# zero-width
In general how satisfying do you find the way you are spending your life these days. Would you call it.....?					
Completely satisfying	O-SLL-c-sq-v-3-a (261)	10.0			23
Pretty satisfying		8.1	1.35	0.08	
Not very satisfying		3.0	1.72	0.11	15
Are you...with the life you lead?					
Very satisfied	O-SLL-u-sq-v-3-a (258)	10.0			9
Fairly satisfied		7.4	1.58	0.10	
Dissatisfied		2.9	1.72	0.11	22
On the whole how satisfied are you with the life you lead?					
Very satisfied	O-SLL-u-sq-v-4-b (247)	10.0			8
Fairly satisfied		7.9	1.13	0.07	
Not very satisfied		4.3	1.45	0.09	
Not at all satisfied		1.6	1.30	0.08	40
I am very happy with the kind of life I lead					
Strongly agree	O-SLL-u-sq-v-5-a (240)	10.0			18
Agree		8.3	1.00	0.06	
Neither agree nor disagree		5.4	1.24	0.08	
Disagree		3.7	1.24	0.08	
Strongly disagree		1.3	1.08	0.07	32

(continued)

Table B.5 (continued)

Item	Question code (valid assessments)	Upper boundary	Standard deviation	Standard error	# zero-width
In general, are you satisfied or dissatisfied with the way things are going in your own personal life?					
Satisfied	O-SLP-g-sq-v-2-b (243)	10.0			–
Dissatisfied		4.7	1.66	0.11	
How satisfied are you with the way you are getting on now?					
Very satisfied	O-SLS-c-sq-v-3-aa (254)	10.0			7
All right		6.9	1.69	0.11	
Not at all		2.4	1.60	0.10	23
On the whole, are you...?					
Fully satisfied	O-Slu-u-sq-v-4-b (242)	10.0			25
Not fully but generally satisfied		8.2	1.45	0.09	
Still dissatisfied		4.4	1.47	0.09	
Extremely dissatisfied		1.5	1.29	0.08	27
Are you satisfied with your life?					
Very much	O-Slu-u-sq-v-4-c (249)	10.0			11
Much		7.9	1.22	0.08	
To some extend		4.8	1.54	0.10	
Not at all		1.8	1.51	0.10	36
How satisfied are you with your life in general these days?					
Very satisfied	O-SLW-c-sq-v-5-fb (241)	10.0			9
Fairly satisfied		8.1	1.11	0.07	
Satisfied nor dissatisfied		5.4	1.20	0.08	
Fairly dissatisfied		3.7	1.17	0.08	
Very dissatisfied		1.4	1.04	0.07	25
All things considered, how satisfied are you with your life as-a-whole these days?					
Completely satisfied	O-SLW-c-sq-v-5-p (240)	10.0			43
Very satisfied		8.8	1.13	0.07	
Satisfied		6.3	1.24	0.08	
Not very satisfied		3.8	1.29	0.08	
Not at all satisfied		1.2	1.14	0.07	46

Table B.6 Assessments by 245 American students of items from English11

Item	Question code (valid assessments)	Upper boundary	Standard deviation	Standard error	# zero-width
In general, how satisfied or dissatisfied are you with the way things are going in your personal life at this time? Are you					
Very satisfied	O-SLP-c-sq-v-4-a (232)	10.0			9
Somewhat satisfied		7.9	1.10	0.07	
Somewhat dissatisfied		4.5	1.28	0.08	
Very dissatisfied		1.7	1.11	0.07	24
In general, how satisfied are you with your life?					
Very satisfied	O-SLu-g-sq-v-4-e (219)	10.0			22
Satisfied		8.3	1.31	0.09	
Dissatisfied		5.4	1.43	0.10	
Very dissatisfied		2.0	1.28	0.09	12
How do you feel about your life as a whole right now? Are you satisfied or dissatisfied?					
Strongly satisfied	O-SLW-c-sq-v-4-b (228)	10.0			9
Somewhat satisfied		7.9	1.24	0.08	
Somewhat dissatisfied		4.4	1.31	0.09	
Strongly dissatisfied		1.6	1.16	0.08	18
Please tell me how satisfied you are with your life overall. Would you say that you are					
Very satisfied	O-SLW-g-sq-v-4-b (228)	10.0			9
Mostly satisfied		8.0	1.24	0.08	
Mostly dissatisfied		4.4	1.37	0.09	
Very dissatisfied		1.7	1.17	0.08	18
We'd like to know how satisfied or dissatisfied you are with different aspects of your life. Are you completely satisfied, somewhat satisfied, somewhat dissatisfied, or completely dissatisfied with........Your life as a whole?					
Completely satisfied	O-SLW-u-sq-v-4-e (224)	10.0			29
Somewhat satisfied		8.4	1.34	0.09	
Somewhat dissatisfied		4.5	1.26	0.08	
Completely dissatisfied		1.3	1.22	0.08	39
How satisfied are you with your life in general?					
Very satisfied	O-SLW-u-sq-v-4-d (228)	10.0			9
Somewhat satisfied		7.9	1.26	0.08	
Somewhat dissatisfied		4.4	1.31	0.09	
Very dissatisfied		1.6	1.11	0.07	20

(continued)

Table B.6 (continued)

Item	Question code (valid assessments)	Upper boundary	Standard deviation	Standard error	# zero-width
Overall, how satisfied are you with your present life.......?					
Very satisfied	O-SLu-c-sq-v-5-a (222)	10.0			108
Fairly satisfied		9.2	1.03	0.07	
Neither satisfied nor dissatisfied		6.7	1.25	0.08	
Fairly dissatisfied		4.3	1.32	0.09	
Very dissatisfied		2.2	1.45	0.10	20
Taken all things together, how satisfied are you with your life as a whole these days? On the whole, would you say you are.....?					
Very satisfied	O-SLW-c-sq-v-5-g (219)	10.0			7
Fairly satisfied		8.2	0.88	0.06	
Neither satisfied nor dissatisfied		5.4	1.10	0.07	
Fairly dissatisfied		3.6	1.12	0.08	
Very dissatisfied		1.4	0.96	0.07	22
Now I want to ask you about your life as a whole. How satisfied are you with your life as a whole these days? Which letter on the card comes closest to your feelings?					
Completely satisfied	O-SLW-c-sq-v-5-r (220)	10.0			37
Somewhat satisfied		8.6	1.18	0.08	
Neither satisfied nor dissatisfied		5.5	1.13	0.08	
Somewhat dissatisfied		3.6	1.06	0.07	
Completely dissatisfied		1.0	0.97	0.07	56
How do you feel about your life as a whole......?					
Delighted	O-DT-u-sq-v-7-a (207)	10.0			13
Pleased		8.7	0.72	0.05	
Mostly satisfied		6.7	0.74	0.05	
Mixed		5.1	0.78	0.05	
Mostly dissatisfied		3.7	0.80	0.06	
Unhappy		2.4	0.74	0.05	
Terrible		0.8	0.67	0.05	41

Table B.7 Assessments by 233 American students of items from English12

Item	Question code (valid assessments)	Upper boundary	Standard deviation	Standard error	# zero-width
Taken all together, how would you say things are these days? Would you say that you are....?					
Very happy	O-HL-c-sq-v-3-aa (223)	10.0			5
Pretty happy		7.3	1.40	0.09	
Not too happy		2.5	1.52	0.10	22
Taking all things together, how would you say things are these days? Would you say you are...?					
Very happy	O-HL-c-sq-v-3-ab (225)	10.0			5
Fairly happy		7.3	1.36	0.09	
Not too happy		2.9	1.56	0.10	14
In general, how happy would you say you are?					
Very happy	O-HL-g-sq-v-3-a (223)	10.0			4
Fairly happy		7.4	1.33	0.09	
Not at all happy		2.4	1.53	0.10	18
Generally speaking, how happy would you say you are?					
Very happy	O-HL-g-sq-v-3-k (219)	10.0			4
Somewhat happy		7.2	1.42	0.10	
Not happy		2.7	1.56	0.11	18
In general, how happy would you say you are.....?					
Very happy	O-HL-g-sq-v-3-f (222)	10.0			5
Fairly happy		7.3	1.36	0.09	
Not very happy		2.7	1.58	0.11	23
In general, how happy would you say you are?					
Very happy	O-HL-g-sq-v-3-l (223)	10.0			3
Fairly happy		7.4	1.35	0.09	
Not happy		3.0	1.60	0.11	17
Generally speaking, how happy would you say you are.....?					
Very happy	O-HL-g-sq-v-3-d (223)	10.0			3
Fairly happy		7.2	1.40	0.09	
Not too happy		2.6	1.52	0.10	19
If you were to consider your life in general, how happy or unhappy would you say you are on the whole?					
Very happy	O-HL-g-sq-v-4-g (219)	10.0			4
Fairly happy		7.8	1.07	0.07	
Fairly unhappy		4.3	1.26	0.09	
Very unhappy		1.7	1.06	0.07	21
Would you describe yourself as					
Very happy	O-HP-g-sq-v-4-b (214)	10.0			4
Somewhat happy		7.8	1.04	0.07	
Somewhat unhappy		4.4	1.29	0.09	
Very unhappy		1.7	1.14	0.08	20

(continued)

Table B.7 (continued)

Item	Question code (valid assessments)	Upper boundary	Standard deviation	Standard error	# zero-width
Taking all things together in your life, how would you say things are these days? Would you say you are					
Very happy	O-HL-c-sq-v-5-g (212)	10.0			8
Fairly happy		8.1	0.93	0.06	
Neither happy not unhappy		5.4	1.09	0.07	
Fairly unhappy		3.6	1.02	0.07	
Very unhappy		1.4	0.95	0.07	22

Appendix C: Cumulative Frequencies and Parameters Beta Distributions for Groups of European Countries (Tables C.1, C.2, C.3, C.4, C.5, and C.6)

Table C.1 Cumulative frequencies and parameters beta distribution life satisfaction in Western Europe

Year	Version	On the whole how satisfied are you with the life you lead?				Alpha	Beta	Estimated population mean
		Not at all satisfied	Not very satisfied	Fairly satisfied	Very satisfied			
2004	EB620	2.3%	12.2%	73.4%	100%	3.20	1.52	6.8
2005	EB634	2.4%	13.0%	72.8%	100%	3.05	1.45	6.8
2006	EB652	2.9%	13.7%	73.8%	100%	2.97	1.46	6.7
2007	EB681	2.4%	11.7%	71.3%	100%	3.12	1.42	6.9
2009	EB724	1.9%	11.7%	69.1%	100%	3.06	1.34	7.0
2010	EB734	2.4%	11.8%	69.7%	100%	3.01	1.34	6.9
2011	EB763	2.3%	12.0%	67.9%	100%	2.88	1.25	7.0
2012	EB773	2.0%	8.9%	67.4%	100%	3.31	1.35	7.1
2012	**EB781**	**2.0%**	**9.8%**	**68.1%**	**100%**	**3.22**	**1.35**	**7.0**
2013	EB793	2.1%	8.8%	62.1%	100%	3.00	1.13	7.3
2013	EB801	1.9%	8.8%	62.6%	100%	3.06	1.15	7.3
2014	EB812	1.7%	8.4%	59.6%	100%	2.99	1.07	7.4
2014	EB814	1.3%	6.7%	57.8%	100%	3.31	1.10	7.5
2014	EB823	1.3%	7.6%	60.1%	100%	3.26	1.14	7.4
2015	EB833	1.5%	7.4%	58.8%	100%	3.17	1.09	7.4

Table C.2 Cumulative frequencies and parameters beta distribution satisfaction with democracy in Western Europe

Year	Version	On the whole how satisfied are you with the way the democracy works in your country?				Alpha	Beta	Estimated population mean
		Not at all satisfied	Not very satisfied	Fairly satisfied	Very satisfied			
2004	EB620	7.4%	35.7%	92.2%	100%	3.32	2.80	5.4
2005	EB634	10.5%	40.4%	92.4%	100%	2.83	2.60	5.2
2006	EB652	10.6%	39.8%	92.2%	100%	2.81	2.55	5.2
2007	EB681	7.4%	32.0%	87.0%	100%	2.88	2.17	5.7
2009	EB724	7.6%	35.2%	91.3%	100%	3.18	2.64	5.5
2010	EB734	7.8%	37.1%	91.3%	100%	3.11	2.64	5.4
2011	EB763	7.2%	33.4%	87.5%	100%	2.89	2.22	5.7
2012	EB773	7.1%	30.5%	88.1%	100%	3.06	2.30	5.7
2012	**EB781**	**8.1%**	**32.5%**	**86.6%**	**100%**	**2.73**	**2.07**	**5.7**
2013	EB793	7.5%	29.9%	85.8%	100%	2.82	2.05	5.8
2013	EB801	8.0%	30.8%	84.5%	100%	2.63	1.90	5.8
2014	EB812	6.6%	26.9%	84.6%	100%	2.97	2.03	5.9
2014	EB814	6.8%	27.7%	83.8%	100%	2.83	1.94	5.9
2014	EB823	7.9%	29.5%	85.4%	100%	2.76	1.99	5.8
2015	EB833	6.7%	26.6%	83.2%	100%	2.86	1.91	6.0

Table C.3 Cumulative frequencies and parameters beta distribution life satisfaction in Southern Europe

Year	Version	On the whole how satisfied are you with the life you lead?				Alpha	Beta	Estimated population mean
		Not at all satisfied	Not very satisfied	Fairly satisfied	Very satisfied			
2004	EB620	3.6%	20.8%	80.1%	100%	3.02	0.99	7.5
2005	EB634	4.1%	22.8%	88.6%	100%	3.57	1.36	7.2
2006	EB652	3.7%	19.9%	83.8%	100%	3.38	1.14	7.5
2007	EB681	4.0%	23.5%	85.6%	100%	3.23	1.19	7.3
2009	EB724	6.5%	28.5%	91.4%	100%	3.17	1.42	6.9
2010	EB734	6.6%	28.3%	89.3%	100%	2.94	1.28	7.0
2011	EB763	7.6%	33.8%	93.7%	100%	3.10	1.57	6.6
2012	EB773	10.2%	36.7%	90.4%	100%	2.36	1.23	6.6
2012	**EB781**	**11.1%**	**38.5%**	**91.6%**	**100%**	**2.35**	**1.29**	**6.5**
2013	EB793	13.5%	44.8%	90.1%	100%	1.93	1.16	6.2
2013	EB801	14.1%	42.7%	91.0%	100%	1.97	1.18	6.3
2014	EB812	14.6%	43.5%	89.2%	100%	1.80	1.07	6.3
2014	EB814	8.8%	34.2%	87.0%	100%	2.29	1.08	6.8
2014	EB823	8.4%	34.3%	88.3%	100%	2.43	1.17	6.8
2015	EB833	6.6%	32.4%	88.7%	100%	2.73	1.25	6.9

Table C.4 Cumulative frequencies and parameters beta distribution satisfaction with democracy in Southern Europe

Year	Version	On the whole how satisfied are you with the way the democracy works in your country?				Alpha	Beta	Estimated population mean
		Not at all satisfied	Not very satisfied	Fairly satisfied	Very satisfied			
2004	EB620	11.1%	46.1%	85.0%	100%	1.92	1.53	5.6
2005	EB634	13.8%	46.1%	90.7%	100%	2.03	1.79	5.3
2006	EB652	10.4%	40.6%	87.3%	100%	2.21	1.69	5.7
2007	EB681	12.3%	45.7%	88.3%	100%	2.02	1.69	5.4
2009	EB724	11.5%	50.3%	93.2%	100%	2.42	2.23	5.2
2010	EB734	14.0%	51.3%	90.3%	100%	1.95	1.81	5.2
2011	EB763	20.8%	61.6%	94.8%	100%	1.74	2.08	4.6
2012	EB773	25.2%	69.4%	95.2%	100%	1.56	2.15	4.2
2012	**EB781**	**27.7%**	**71.3%**	**96.3%**	**100%**	**1.52**	**2.24**	**4.0**
2013	EB793	30.8%	75.3%	96.4%	100%	1.42	2.29	3.8
2013	EB801	34.5%	77.2%	96.0%	100%	1.24	2.14	3.7
2014	EB812	31.9%	78.0%	97.8%	100%	1.55	2.66	3.7
2014	EB814	28.3%	71.7%	98.1%	100%	1.66	2.53	4.0
2014	EB823	32.7%	74.2%	98.3%	100%	1.46	2.44	3.7
2015	EB833	25.3%	69.0%	97.4%	100%	1.73	2.45	4.1

Table C.5 Cumulative frequencies and parameters beta distribution life satisfaction in Eastern Europe

Year	Version	On the whole how satisfied are you with the life you lead?				Alpha	Beta	Estimated population mean
		Not at all satisfied	Not very satisfied	Fairly satisfied	Very satisfied			
2004	EB620	6.8%	30.3%	86.9%	100%	2.12	1.17	6.4
2005	EB634	6.3%	29.8%	85.8%	100%	2.11	1.13	6.5
2006	EB652	5.4%	28.6%	88.0%	100%	2.39	1.28	6.5
2007	EB681	4.8%	25.3%	85.1%	100%	2.38	1.15	6.7
2009	EB724	7.1%	27.1%	87.6%	100%	2.23	1.19	6.5
2010	EB734	5.1%	24.4%	85.7%	100%	2.42	1.17	6.7
2011	EB763	5.7%	27.7%	89.3%	100%	2.49	1.35	6.5
2012	EB773	6.5%	27.2%	88.0%	100%	2.32	1.24	6.5
2012	**EB781**	**5.9%**	**26.6%**	**89.9%**	**100%**	**2.55**	**1.38**	**6.5**
2013	EB793	6.4%	29.5%	88.2%	100%	2.28	1.26	6.4
2013	EB801	6.3%	29.9%	89.0%	100%	2.32	1.30	6.4
2014	EB812	6.2%	29.2%	87.0%	100%	2.22	1.20	6.5
2014	EB814	5.0%	24.4%	83.8%	100%	2.30	1.09	6.8
2014	EB823	4.6%	24.1%	84.8%	100%	2.43	1.15	6.8
2015	EB833	4.2%	23.4%	84.8%	100%	2.51	1.16	6.8

Table C.6 Cumulative frequencies and parameters beta distribution satisfaction with democracy in Eastern Europe

Year	Version	On the whole how satisfied are you with the way the democracy works in your country? Not at all satisfied	Not very satisfied	Fairly satisfied	Very satisfied	Alpha	Beta	Estimated population mean
2004	EB620	19.5%	63.1%	96.7%	100%	1.89	2.19	4.6
2005	EB634	22.8%	65.3%	97.2%	100%	1.74	2.17	4.4
2006	EB652	16.7%	56.6%	95.1%	100%	1.89	1.92	5.0
2007	EB681	12.9%	54.7%	96.2%	100%	2.35	2.26	5.1
2009	EB724	17.2%	57.5%	96.0%	100%	1.95	2.04	4.9
2010	EB734	11.8%	50.1%	96.5%	100%	2.49	2.26	5.2
2011	EB763	15.0%	51.3%	95.1%	100%	2.03	1.90	5.2
2012	EB773	18.7%	57.8%	96.6%	100%	1.89	2.04	4.8
2012	**EB781**	**17.3%**	**59.2%**	**96.4%**	**100%**	**1.99**	**2.14**	**4.8**
2013	EB793	24.7%	67.3%	97.4%	100%	1.67	2.19	4.3
2013	EB801	23.2%	65.9%	96.2%	100%	1.62	2.02	4.5
2014	EB812	19.5%	63.6%	97.0%	100%	1.93	2.26	4.6
2014	EB814	19.5%	60.7%	97.3%	100%	1.92	2.19	4.7
2014	EB823	21.5%	59.9%	97.4%	100%	1.78	2.07	4.6
2015	EB833	18.3%	58.3%	96.7%	100%	1.93	2.09	4.8

Appendix D: Horizontal and Vertical Deviation of Reference Boundaries for Groups of European Countries

The values of the horizontal and vertical deviations depicted in Figs. 9.3 and 9.4 are given in the tables in this appendix. The fixed reference boundaries for the response options of the Eurobarometer item and derived from the beta distribution that best fits the 2012-wave of European Social Survey are given in each table. The response option 'Very satisfied' has been omitted from each table, as the reference boundary for this option is by definition equal to 10. The horizontal deviations for each wave of the Eurobarometer are given in the columns below the reference boundaries. The vertical deviations to the cumulative frequencies for each wave are given in the following three columns. A reference to the table in which the cumulative frequency distributions can be found is given above the columns with the vertical deviations for these cumulative frequencies.

Illustration Horizontal Deviation The reference boundary for the response option 'Not very satisfied' in Table D.1 is equal to 4.23. This horizontal deviation of this reference boundary for the 2005 wave is equal to −0.06. This means that the beta distribution that best fits the fixed boundaries and the cumulative frequencies of this 2005 wave is equal to the cumulative frequency for the response option 'Not very satisfied' at a value of 4.29 on the 0–10 continuum.

Table D.1 Horizontal and vertical deviation for life satisfaction in Western Europe

		On the whole how satisfied are you with the life you lead?					
		Not at all satisfied	Not very satisfied	Fairly satisfied	Not at all satisfied	Not very satisfied	Fairly satisfied
Reference boundaries		2.52	4.23	8.28	See Table C.1 for cumulative frequencies		
Year	Version	Horizontal deviation			Vertical deviation		
2004	EB620	0.07	−0.03	0.01	−0.21% pts	0.28% pts	−0.10% pts
2005	EB634	0.12	−0.06	0.01	−0.38% pts	0.50% pts	−0.21% pts
2006	EB652	0.06	−0.03	0.00	−0.22% pts	0.30% pts	−0.08% pts
2007	EB681	0.04	−0.02	0.00	−0.12% pts	0.15% pts	−0.06% pts
2009	EB724	0.17	−0.08	0.01	−0.46% pts	0.61% pts	−0.22% pts
2010	EB734	0.07	−0.04	0.00	−0.20% pts	0.28% pts	−0.09% pts
2011	EB763	0.14	−0.07	0.01	−0.40% pts	0.53% pts	−0.19% pts
2012	EB773	−0.12	0.05	−0.01	0.28% pts	−0.34% pts	0.11% pts
2012	**EB781**	**0.00**	**0.00**	**0.00**	**0.00% pts**	**0.00% pts**	**−0.01% pts**
2013	EB793	−0.05	0.02	0.00	0.11% pts	−0.15% pts	0.05% pts
2013	EB801	−0.02	0.01	0.00	0.06% pts	−0.09% pts	0.05% pts
2014	EB812	0.03	−0.01	0.00	−0.05% pts	0.04% pts	−0.05% pts
2014	EB814	−0.05	−0.01	0.00	0.08% pts	0.05% pts	0.08% pts
2014	EB823	0.03	−0.04	0.00	−0.06% pts	0.23% pts	−0.01% pts
2015	EB833	−0.02	0.00	0.00	0.04% pts	0.02% pts	0.03% pts

Illustration Vertical Deviation It can be seen from Table C.1 that the cumulative frequency for the response option 'Not very satisfied' is equal to 13.0%. The vertical deviation for this response option in the 2005 wave is according to Table D.1 equal to 0.50 pts. This means that value of the beta distribution that best fits the fixed boundaries and the cumulative frequencies of the 2005 wave is 12.5% at the reference boundary for the response option 'Not very satisfied' (Tables D.2, D.3, D.4, D.5, and D.6).

Table D.2 Horizontal and vertical deviation for satisfaction with democracy in Western Europe

		On the whole how satisfied are you with the way the democracy works in your country?					
		Not at all satisfied	Not very satisfied	Fairly satisfied	Not at all satisfied	Not very satisfied	Fairly satisfied
Reference boundaries		2.60	4.70	8.10	See Table C.2 for cumulative frequencies		
Year	Version	Horizontal deviation			Vertical deviation		
2004	EB620	0.01	−0.01	0.00	0.0% pts	0.1% pts	0.0% pts
2005	EB634	0.00	0.00	0.00	0.0% pts	0.1% pts	0.0% pts
2006	EB652	−0.01	0.01	−0.01	0.1% pts	−0.2% pts	0.1% pts
2007	EB681	0.02	−0.01	0.01	−0.1% pts	0.2% pts	−0.1% pts
2009	EB724	0.01	−0.01	0.00	0.0% pts	0.1% pts	0.0% pts
2010	EB734	0.05	−0.05	0.03	−0.4% pts	0.8% pts	−0.3% pts
2011	EB763	0.06	−0.05	0.03	−0.5% pts	0.8% pts	−0.3% pts
2012	EB773	−0.05	0.04	−0.02	0.3% pts	−0.6% pts	0.2% pts
2012	**EB781**	**0.00**	**0.00**	**0.00**	**0.0% pts**	**0.0% pts**	**0.0% pts**
2013	EB793	−0.04	0.04	−0.02	0.3% pts	−0.6% pts	0.2% pts
2013	EB801	−0.01	0.01	0.00	0.1% pts	−0.2% pts	0.1% pts
2014	EB812	−0.09	0.07	−0.03	0.6% pts	−1.0% pts	0.4% pts
2014	EB814	−0.05	0.04	−0.02	0.3% pts	−0.6% pts	0.2% pts
2014	EB823	−0.07	0.07	−0.03	0.5% pts	−1.0% pts	0.4% pts
2015	EB833	−0.08	0.07	−0.02	0.5% pts	−0.9% pts	0.3% pts

Table D.3 Horizontal and vertical deviation for life satisfaction in Southern Europe

		On the whole how satisfied are you with the life you lead?					
		Not at all satisfied	Not very satisfied	Fairly satisfied	Not at all satisfied	Not very satisfied	Fairly satisfied
Reference boundaries		3.38	5.96	9.31	See Table C.3 for cumulative frequencies		
Year	Version	Horizontal deviation			Vertical deviation		
2004	EB620	0.02	−0.02	0.00	−0.1% pts	0.2% pts	0.0% pts
2005	EB634	−0.14	0.07	−0.02	0.5% pts	−0.9% pts	0.3% pts
2006	EB652	−0.14	0.06	−0.01	0.5% pts	−0.7% pts	0.4% pts
2007	EB681	0.00	0.00	0.00	0.0% pts	0.0% pts	0.0% pts
2009	EB724	−0.15	0.10	−0.03	0.8% pts	−1.4% pts	0.5% pts
2010	EB734	−0.10	0.08	−0.02	0.5% pts	−1.0% pts	0.3% pts
2011	EB763	−0.08	0.06	−0.02	0.5% pts	−0.9% pts	0.3% pts
2012	EB773	0.01	−0.01	0.00	0.0% pts	0.1% pts	0.0% pts
2012	**EB781**	**0.00**	**0.00**	**0.00**	**0.0% pts**	**0.0% pts**	**0.0% pts**

(continued)

Table D.3 (continued)

		On the whole how satisfied are you with the life you lead?					
		Not at all satisfied	Not very satisfied	Fairly satisfied	Not at all satisfied	Not very satisfied	Fairly satisfied
Reference boundaries		3.38	5.96	9.31	See Table C.3 for cumulative frequencies		
Year	Version	Horizontal deviation			Vertical deviation		
2013	EB793	0.15	−0.20	0.06	−1.2% pts	2.6% pts	−0.9% pts
2013	EB801	0.04	−0.05	0.02	−0.3% pts	0.7% pts	−0.2% pts
2014	EB812	0.09	−0.13	0.04	−0.7% pts	1.7% pts	−0.6% pts
2014	EB814	0.08	−0.08	0.02	−0.5% pts	1.0% pts	−0.4% pts
2014	EB823	0.07	−0.07	0.02	−0.4% pts	0.9% pts	−0.3% pts
2015	EB833	0.11	−0.08	0.02	−0.6% pts	1.1% pts	−0.4% pts

Table D.4 Horizontal and vertical deviation for satisfaction with democracy in Southern Europe

		On the whole how satisfied are you with the way the democracy works in your country?					
		Not at all satisfied	Not very satisfied	Fairly satisfied	Not at all satisfied	Not very satisfied	Fairly satisfied
Reference boundaries		2.39	5.40	8.25	See Table C.4 for cumulative frequencies		
Year	Version	Horizontal deviation			Vertical deviation		
2004	EB620	0.00	0.00	0.00	0.0% pts	0.0% pts	0.0% pts
2005	EB634	−0.18	0.29	−0.17	1.8% pts	−4.2% pts	1.8% pts
2006	EB652	−0.19	0.25	−0.12	1.5% pts	−3.6% pts	1.5% pts
2007	EB681	−0.11	0.17	−0.09	1.0% pts	−2.4% pts	1.0% pts
2009	EB724	−0.10	0.14	−0.11	1.0% pts	−2.3% pts	1.0% pts
2010	EB734	−0.05	0.09	−0.05	0.5% pts	−1.3% pts	0.5% pts
2011	EB763	−0.05	0.12	−0.11	0.6% pts	−1.6% pts	0.7% pts
2012	EB773	0.02	−0.05	0.05	−0.2% pts	0.6% pts	−0.3% pts
2012	**EB781**	**0.00**	**0.00**	**0.00**	**0.0% pts**	**0.0% pts**	**0.0% pts**
2013	EB793	0.03	−0.10	0.12	−0.4% pts	1.1% pts	−0.5% pts
2013	EB801	0.03	−0.15	0.17	−0.5% pts	1.5% pts	−0.7% pts
2014	EB812	0.01	−0.04	0.07	−0.2% pts	0.5% pts	−0.2% pts
2014	EB814	−0.04	0.14	−0.24	0.7% pts	−1.8% pts	0.8% pts
2014	EB823	−0.04	0.15	−0.26	0.6% pts	−1.8% pts	0.8% pts
2015	EB833	−0.04	0.12	−0.18	0.6% pts	−1.7% pts	0.7% pts

Table D.5 Horizontal and vertical deviation for life satisfaction in Eastern Europe

		On the whole how satisfied are you with the life you lead?					
		Not at all satisfied	Not very satisfied	Fairly satisfied	Not at all satisfied	Not very satisfied	Fairly satisfied
Reference boundaries		2.74	5.11	9.14	See Table C.5 for cumulative frequencies		
Year	Version	Horizontal deviation			Vertical deviation		
2004	EB620	0.18	−0.16	0.04	−1.1% pts	1.8% pts	−0.6% pts
2005	EB634	0.23	−0.20	0.05	−1.3% pts	2.2% pts	−0.8% pts
2006	EB652	0.20	−0.15	0.04	−1.1% pts	1.8% pts	−0.6% pts
2007	EB681	0.19	−0.13	0.03	−0.9% pts	1.4% pts	−0.6% pts
2009	EB724	−0.01	0.01	0.00	0.0% pts	−0.1% pts	0.1% pts
2010	EB734	0.07	−0.05	0.01	−0.3% pts	0.6% pts	−0.2% pts
2011	EB763	0.09	−0.07	0.02	−0.5% pts	0.8% pts	−0.3% pts
2012	EB773	0.03	−0.03	0.01	−0.2% pts	0.3% pts	−0.1% pts
2012	**EB781**	**0.00**	**0.00**	**0.00**	**0.0% pts**	**0.0% pts**	**0.0% pts**
2013	EB793	0.15	−0.12	0.03	−0.8% pts	1.4% pts	−0.5% pts
2013	EB801	0.14	−0.12	0.03	−0.8% pts	1.5% pts	−0.5% pts
2014	EB812	0.18	−0.15	0.04	−1.0% pts	1.7% pts	−0.6% pts
2014	EB814	0.14	−0.10	0.02	−0.6% pts	1.1% pts	−0.4% pts
2014	EB823	0.15	−0.10	0.02	−0.7% pts	1.1% pts	−0.4% pts
2015	EB833	0.15	−0.10	0.02	−0.6% pts	1.1% pts	−0.4% pts

Table D.6 Horizontal and vertical deviation for satisfaction with democracy in Eastern Europe

		On the whole how satisfied are you with the way the democracy works in your country?					
		Not at all satisfied	Not very satisfied	Fairly satisfied	Not at all satisfied	Not very satisfied	Fairly satisfied
Reference boundaries		2.51	5.40	8.70	See Table C.6 for cumulative frequencies		
Year	Version	Horizontal deviation			Vertical deviation		
2004	EB620	0.02	−0.04	0.05	−0.3% pts	0.6% pts	−0.3% pts
2005	EB634	0.00	0.00	0.01	0.0% pts	0.1% pts	0.0% pts
2006	EB652	0.00	−0.01	0.00	0.0% pts	0.1% pts	0.0% pts
2007	EB681	0.00	0.00	0.00	0.0% pts	−0.1% pts	0.0% pts
2009	EB724	−0.02	0.03	−0.03	0.2% pts	−0.5% pts	0.2% pts
2010	EB734	−0.08	0.11	−0.11	0.8% pts	−1.8% pts	0.7% pts
2011	EB763	−0.08	0.12	−0.09	0.8% pts	−1.8% pts	0.7% pts
2012	EB773	−0.05	0.10	−0.10	0.6% pts	−1.4% pts	0.6% pts
2012	**EB781**	**0.00**	**0.00**	**0.00**	**0.0% pts**	**0.0% pts**	**0.0% pts**
2013	EB793	0.00	−0.01	0.02	−0.1% pts	0.2% pts	−0.1% pts
2013	EB801	0.04	−0.09	0.10	−0.5% pts	1.2% pts	−0.5% pts
2014	EB812	0.02	−0.03	0.04	−0.2% pts	0.5% pts	−0.2% pts
2014	EB814	−0.03	0.07	−0.08	0.4% pts	−1.0% pts	0.4% pts
2014	EB823	−0.07	0.15	−0.17	0.9% pts	−2.2% pts	0.9% pts
2015	EB833	−0.04	0.08	−0.08	0.5% pts	−1.1% pts	0.5% pts

Appendix E: Cumulative Distributions and Parameters Beta Distribution

E.1: Cumulative Frequencies and Parameters Beta Distribution USA (Tables E.1.1, E.1.2, E.1.3, E.1.4, E.1.5, E.1.6, and E.1.7)

Table E.1.1 Cumulative frequencies O-SLP-g-sq-v-2-b, Gallup Poll

	In general, are you satisfied or dissatisfied with the way things are going in your own personal life?	
Year	Dissatisfied	Satisfied
1973	21.3%	100%
1979	21.6%	100%
1981	17.1%	100%

(continued)

Table E.1.1 (continued)

Year	In general, are you satisfied or dissatisfied with the way things are going in your own personal life?	
	Dissatisfied	Satisfied
1982	23.2%	100%
1983	21.5%	100%
1984	18.5%	100%
1985	16.6%	100%
1986	14.7%	100%
1987	15.1%	100%
1988	14.4%	100%
1990	14.4%	100%
1991	15.4%	100%
1992	21.2%	100%
1993	17.2%	100%
1996	12.2%	100%
1997	14.4%	100%
1998	13.5%	100%
2000	12.1%	100%
2001	14.1%	100%
2006	15.2%	100%
2008	18.7%	100%

Table E.1.2 Cumulative frequencies O-SLP-c-sq-v-2-a, Gallup Poll

Year	In general, are you satisfied with the way things are going in your personal life at this time?	
	Dissatisfied	Satisfied
2001	15.4%	100%
2002	14.9%	100%
2003	12.5%	100%
2004	13.9%	100%
2007	14.3%	100%
2011	21.2%	100%
2013	20.2%	100%

Table E.1.3 Cumulative frequencies and parameters beta distribution O-SLP-c-sq-v-4-a, Gallup

Year	In general, how satisfied or dissatisfied are you with the way things are going in your personal life at this time? Are you a person who has all the bad things in his life? Other circles are in between. Which circle do you think comes closest to matching your life?				Parameters best fit beta distribution	
	Very dissatisfied	Somewhat dissatisfied	Somewhat satisfied	Very satisfied	α	ß
2001	4.7%	15.0%	45.4%	100%	5.56	2.68
2002	5.1%	15.2%	46.5%	100%	5.54	2.72
2003	4.5%	12.6%	41.4%	100%	5.36	2.40
2004	5.1%	14.3%	40.8%	100%	***4.72***	***2.09***

Table E.1.4 Cumulative frequencies and parameters beta distribution O-SLu-u-sq-v-4-f, Gallup

Year	Overall, how satisfied are you with your life.....?				Parameters best fit beta distribution	
	Very dissatisfied	Somewhat dissatisfied	Somewhat satisfied	Very satisfied	α	ß
2005	3.6%	11.5%	49.9%	100%	**4.72**	**2.09**
2007	2.7%	8.3%	42.6%	100%	4.84	1.86
2008	4.8%	13.6%	53.5%	100%	***4.44***	***2.12***

Table E.1.5 Cumulative frequencies and parameters beta distribution O-SLu-g-sq-v-4-e, BRFSS

Year	In general, how satisfied are you with your life? Would you say you are				Parameters best fit beta distribution	
	Very dissatisfied	Somewhat dissatisfied	Somewhat satisfied	Very satisfied	α	ß
2005	1.1%	5.6%	55.4%	100%	4.35	2.11
2006	1.0%	5.0%	54.3%	100%	***4.52***	***2.14***
2007	1.1%	5.5%	55.6%	100%	4.40	2.14
2008	1.0%	5.2%	54.6%	100%	**4.44**	**2.12**
2009	1.1%	5.9%	55.4%	100%	4.29	2.09
2010	1.0%	5.4%	54.1%	100%	4.35	2.06
2013	1.3%	6.6%	54.1%	100%	–	–
2014	0.8%	4.1%	50.7%	100%	–	–

Table E.1.6 Cumulative frequencies and parameters beta distribution O-SLu-g-sq-v-4-da, LAPOP

Year	In general, how satisfied are you with your life? Would you say you are				Parameters best fit beta distribution	
	Very dissatisfied	Somewhat dissatisfied	Somewhat satisfied	Very satisfied	α	ß
2008	6.1%	24.2%	73.7%	100%	***4.44***	***2.12***
2010	4.9%	19.5%	69.2%	100%	4.65	2.00
2012	4.0%	19.5%	70.1%	100%	5.03	2.16

Table E.1.7 Cumulative frequencies and parameters beta distribution O-SLW-c-sq-n-10-a, WVS

	All things considered, how satisfied are you with your life as-a-whole now.....?										Parameters best fit beta distribution	
Year	Dissatisfied	2	3	4	5	6	7	8	9	Satisfied	α	ß
1982	0.8%	2.0%	3.8%	7.2%	15.5%	22.8%	37.8%	61.5%	81.7%	100%	3.08	1.23
1990	0.6%	1.4%	3.3%	5.6%	12.7%	19.5%	34.5%	62.6%	84.1%	100%	3.76	1.45
1995	0.9%	2.2%	3.9%	6.7%	14.6%	22.1%	37.6%	63.3%	81.4%	100%	3.10	1.24
1999	0.9%	1.4%	3.3%	5.9%	13.0%	21.3%	39.7%	64.9%	84.1%	100%	3.57	1.44
2006	0.5%	1.4%	3.4%	7.3%	14.6%	24.3%	47.4%	75.6%	93.3%	100%	**4.52**	**2.14**
2011	1.2%	2.5%	5.0%	9.6%	16.8%	24.1%	41.3%	71.7%	90.7%	100%	3.44	1.62

E.2: Cumulative Frequencies and Parameters Beta Distribution Japan (Tables E.2.1, E.2.2, E.2.3, E.2.4, E.2.5, E.2.6, E.2.7, and E.2.8)

Table E.2.1 Cumulative frequencies and parameters beta distribution O-SLu-c-sq-v-4-f, LIN

	By the way, how do you feel about your life?				Parameters best fit beta distribution	
Year	I cannot stand my current life	My current life is far from satisfactory	I am not satisfied with my current life, but it is not too bad to keep more or less on the current level	My life could be better, but on the whole I am satisfied with my current life	α	ß
1958	9.2%	38.8%	83.7%	100%	3.58	1.96
1959	6.7%	31.9%	82.4%	100%	4.26	2.08
1961	5.6%	35.8%	85.5%	100%	4.72	2.44
1962	5.3%	36.1%	83.5%	100%	4.50	2.28
1963	5.1%	32.7%	80.6%	100%	***4.37***	***2.08***

Table E.2.2 Cumulative frequencies and parameters beta distribution O-SLu-u-sq-v-4-e, LIN

	How do you feel about your life?				Parameters best fit beta distribution	
Year	Extremely dissatisfied	Fairly dissatisfied	Rather satisfied, but not sufficiently	Sufficiently satisfied	α	ß
1964	3.5%	37.7%	95.5%	100%	**4.37**	**2.08**
1965	4.3%	38.7%	95.4%	100%	4.11	2.00
1966	5.0%	40.2%	95.4%	100%	3.88	1.95
1967	4.3%	38.1%	94.7%	100%	3.97	1.89
1968	4.1%	34.5%	93.7%	100%	3.98	1.78
1969	4.1%	35.5%	94.2%	100%	***4.04***	***1.84***

Table E.2.3 Cumulative frequencies and parameters beta distribution O-SLu-c-sq-v-4-e, LIN

	How do you feel with life these days?				Parameters best fit beta distribution	
Year	Very dissatisfied	Somewhat dissatisfied	Somewhat satisfied	Very satisfied	α	ß
1970	3.9%	33.8%	93.9%	100%	**4.04**	**1.84**
1971	4.9%	41.5%	95.1%	100%	3.79	1.98
1972	4.6%	39.8%	94.5%	100%	3.79	1.91
1973	5.6%	38.5%	89.8%	100%	2.97	1.40
1974	8.1%	48.7%	96.1%	100%	3.33	2.02
1975	4.8%	38.8%	94.4%	100%	3.75	1.87
1976	4.6%	38.2%	94.1%	100%	3.75	1.84

(continued)

Table E.2.3 (continued)

Year	How do you feel with life these days?				Parameters best fit beta distribution	
	Very dissatisfied	Somewhat dissatisfied	Somewhat satisfied	Very satisfied	α	ß
1977	4.8%	34.9%	90.8%	100%	3.33	1.50
1978	3.9%	34.9%	94.5%	100%	4.12	1.93
1979	3.1%	31.9%	92.8%	100%	4.12	1.78
1980	4.6%	36.6%	94.5%	100%	3.89	1.88
1981	4.6%	35.4%	94.5%	100%	3.94	1.87
1982	4.0%	33.4%	94.2%	100%	4.09	1.87
1983	4.0%	34.5%	94.1%	100%	4.01	1.86
1984	3.9%	34.0%	94.1%	100%	4.07	1.87
1985	3.6%	28.8%	92.6%	100%	4.14	1.73
1986	4.0%	31.2%	93.7%	100%	4.10	1.81
1987	4.1%	34.9%	94.0%	100%	3.94	1.83
1988	4.1%	34.8%	93.7%	100%	3.90	1.81
1989	5.2%	36.3%	94.5%	100%	3.78	1.84
1990	4.3%	32.5%	92.8%	100%	***3.81***	***1.69***
1991	3.7%	32.4%	93.2%	100%	4.02	1.78

Table E.2.4 Cumulative frequencies and parameters beta distribution O-SLW-c-sq-v-4-e, LIN

Year	In general, how satisfied are you with your life? Would you say you are				Parameters best fit beta distribution	
	Very dissatisfied	Somewhat dissatisfied	Somewhat satisfied	Very satisfied	α	ß
1992	6.5%	28.3%	90.4%	100%	4.93	2.27
1993	6.6%	28.1%	89.4%	100%	4.75	2.16
1994	8%	32.2%	91.4%	100%	4.59	2.27
1995	4.9%	25.3%	89.3%	100%	**5.36**	**2.31**
1996	6.3%	28.5%	89.5%	100%	4.81	2.19
1997	8%	31.5%	89.9%	100%	4.36	2.11
1999	10.6%	34.9%	90.3%	100%	**3.83**	**1.99**
2001	10.4%	37.1%	91.7%	100%	4.02	2.17
2002	11%	37.7%	91.9%	100%	**3.95**	**2.16**
2003	11.8%	40.5%	92.6%	100%	3.88	2.22
2004	10.8%	38.4%	92.6%	100%	4.07	2.26
2005	10.8%	38.7%	92.1%	100%	***3.97***	***2.19***
2006	7.5%	32.8%	90.5%	100%	4.51	2.22
2007	9.5%	36.5%	91.6%	100%	4.17	2.21
2008	10.3%	38.9%	91.9%	100%	4.02	2.21
2009	9.8%	38.2%	91.5%	100%	4.05	2.19
2010	9.4%	35.4%	90.8%	100%	4.09	2.12
2011	7.6%	33.6%	89.6%	100%	4.30	2.11

Table E.2.5 Cumulative frequencies and parameters beta distribution O-SLu-c-sq-v-5-n, EAVS

	Overall, to what degree are you satisfied with your life these days?					Parameters best fit beta distribution	
Year	Dissatisfied	Somewhat dissatisfied	Neither satisfied nor dissatisfied	Somewhat satisfied	Satisfied	α	ß
1988	2.7%	12.3%	25.6%	67.1%	100%	3.61	1.83
2002	2.4%	10.7%	25.7%	66.2%	100%	3.75	1.86
2005	2.9%	11.7%	29.3%	72.4%	100%	***3.97***	***2.19***

Table E.2.6 Cumulative frequencies and parameters beta distribution O-SLu-g-sq-v-5-e, LPS

	How satisfied or dissatisfied are you with your life in general?					Parameters best fit beta distribution	
Year	Dissatisfied	Rather dissatisfied	Neither satisfied nor dissatisfied	Somewhat satisfied	Satisfied	α	ß
1978	5.1%	15.8%	42.6%	89.0%	100%	4.01	1.63
1981	5.3%	16.3%	43.5%	89.4%	100%	3.97	1.64
1984	3.5%	15.1%	35.6%	86.3%	100%	4.15	1.50
1987	5.3%	20.0%	50.1%	89.9%	100%	3.75	1.69
1990	5.4%	20.5%	46.3%	90.8%	100%	**3.81**	**1.69**
1993	4.6%	20.4%	48.0%	93.0%	100%	4.27	1.95
1995	4.8%	16.4%	40.0%	85.9%	100%	3.68	1.42
1996	6.5%	22.6%	52.4%	92.3%	100%	3.72	1.81
1999	7.4%	24.1%	55.8%	94.1%	100%	3.81	1.98
2002	7.2%	26.6%	58.7%	95.3%	100%	**3.94**	**2.16**

Table E.2.7 Cumulative frequencies and parameters beta distribution O-SLu-g-sq-v-5-e, FLS

	How satisfied are you with your current life as a whole?					Parameters best fit beta distribution	
Year	Dissatisfied	Somewhat dissatisfied	Neither satisfied nor dissatisfied	Fairly satisfied	Satisfied	α	ß
1995	2.8%	12.4%	34.8%	89.8%	100%	3.98	1.73
1997	2.9%	12.3%	34.9%	90.6%	100%	4.07	1.79
1999	3.5%	16.3%	45.4%	93.2%	100%	***3.83***	***1.99***

Table E.2.8 Cumulative frequencies and parameters beta distribution O-SLW-c-sq-n-10-a, WVS

	All things considered, how satisfied are you with your life as-a-whole now.....?										Parameters best fit beta distribution	
Year	Dissatisfied	2	3	4	5	6	7	8	9	Satisfied	α	ß
1981	1.2%	2.6%	7.0%	12.6%	24.4%	46.2%	65.1%	86.1%	95.4%	100%	5.48	2.38
1990	0.9%	1.9%	5.8%	12.0%	25.3%	47.0%	67.0%	90.8%	96.6%	100%	6.31	2.81
1995	1.6%	3.1%	6.9%	11.3%	25.7%	45.7%	63.2%	87.2%	94.7%	100%	***5.36***	***2.31***
2000	1.7%	3.8%	8.7%	15.0%	28.3%	46.9%	63.5%	88.4%	95.3%	100%	5.00	2.26
2005	0.9%	2%	5.8%	9.4%	17.9%	33.7%	54.0%	81.9%	95.4%	100%	**3.97**	**2.19**
2010	1.3%	2.5%	6.0%	12.0%	24.4%	35.7%	54.5%	80.6%	91.9%	100%	3.13	1.78

E.3: Cumulative Frequencies and Parameters Beta Distribution The Netherlands (Tables E.3.1, E.3.2, E.3.3, E.3.4, E.3.5, and E.3.6)

Table E.3.1 Cumulative frequencies and parameters beta distribution O-SLL-u-sq-v-4-b, EB

	On the whole how satisfied are you with the life you lead?				Parameters best fit beta distribution	
Year	Not at all satisfied	Not very satisfied	Fairly satisfied	Very satisfied	α	ß
1973	0.7%	6.9%	60.5%	100%	7.74	3.31
1975	2.1%	8.4%	64.6%	100%	7.26	3.34
1976	1.5%	8.7%	59.6%	100%	6.70	2.88
1977	1.8%	7.7%	59.6%	100%	**6.88**	**2.94**
1978	1.1%	6.3%	54.9%	100%	7.17	2.83
1979	0.4%	4.3%	54.5%	100%	8.42	3.23
1980	0.4%	5.1%	53.2%	100%	7.76	2.95
1981	1.6%	6.9%	55.8%	100%	6.70	2.69
1982	0.8%	5.9%	53.7%	100%	7.20	2.81
1983	1.3%	6.7%	60.1%	100%	7.61	3.24
1984	0.8%	5.7%	53.6%	100%	7.23	2.82
1985	2.2%	9.3%	63.0%	100%	6.79	3.08
1986	1.4%	7.3%	62.4%	100%	**7.51**	**3.32**
1987	1.2%	7.7%	61.2%	100%	7.35	3.20
1988	1.5%	6.7%	56.1%	100%	6.80	2.73
1989	0.8%	5.3%	54.0%	100%	7.53	2.90
1990	0.8%	6.2%	55.3%	100%	7.44	2.94
1991	0.7%	5.1%	51.0%	100%	7.26	2.67
1992	1.0%	6.2%	50.7%	100%	6.72	2.50
1993	0.8%	5.8%	53.7%	100%	**7.22**	**2.82**
1994	1.3%	7.1%	57.0%	100%	7.06	2.89
1995	1.5%	6.7%	52.3%	100%	6.37	2.44
1997	0.8%	7.2%	53.5%	100%	6.70	2.61
1998	0.9%	5.4%	56.3%	100%	7.86	3.15
1999	0.6%	4.5%	58.7%	100%	8.88	3.61
2000	1.1%	7.1%	61.7%	100%	7.74	3.38
2001	0.9%	5.6%	51.1%	100%	6.98	2.60
2002	1.1%	7.2%	59.4%	100%	7.31	3.11
2003	1.6%	9.8%	60.4%	100%	6.45	2.84
2004	2.0%	7.7%	56.2%	100%	6.30	2.57
2005	0.5%	4.7%	53.1%	100%	7.88	2.98
2006	1.1%	4.9%	52.9%	100%	***7.64***	***2.90***
2007	0.5%	4.0%	48.8%	100%	7.81	2.78
2008	0.4%	3.0%	47.3%	100%	8.67	3.00
2009	0.5%	4.4%	49.4%	100%	7.62	2.74

(continued)

Table E.3.1 (continued)

	On the whole how satisfied are you with the life you lead?				Parameters best fit beta distribution	
Year	Not at all satisfied	Not very satisfied	Fairly satisfied	Very satisfied	α	ß
2010	0.6%	5.0%	49.6%	100%	7.24	2.63
2011	0.8%	4.2%	47.2%	100%	7.31	2.53
2012	1.2%	5.7%	49.2%	100%	6.49	2.35
2013	1.3%	5.3%	54.1%	100%	7.29	2.82
2014	0.5%	5.4%	49.6%	100%	7.14	2.60
2015	0.6%	4.2%	47.5%	100%	7.28	2.53

Table E.3.2 Cumulative frequencies and parameters beta distribution O-SLL-c-sq-v-5-d, CBS

	How satisfied are you with your current life as a whole?					Parameters best fit beta distribution	
Year	Not very satisfied	Fairly satisfied	Satisfied	Very satisfied	Extraordinary satisfied	α	ß
1974	6.0%	19.1%	62.5%	91.9%	100%	7.27	3.00
1977	7.0%	20.7%	65.8%	91.5%	100%	***6.88***	***2.94***
1980	6.6%	17.2%	58.2%	88.4%	100%	6.12	2.64
1983	4.7%	19.1%	66.4%	93.0%	100%	7.74	3.64
1986	4.9%	16.9%	61.3%	91.5%	100%	***7.51***	***3.32***
1989	4.1%	14.1%	45.8%	82.1%	100%	6.19	2.40
1990	3.8%	13.7%	47.2%	83.8%	100%	6.59	2.60
1991	4.3%	12.6%	46.4%	83.4%	100%	6.59	2.57
1992	4.1%	13.0%	47.2%	84.1%	100%	6.69	2.64
1993	3.8%	12.2%	45.9%	84.2%	100%	***7.22***	***2.82***
1994	6.2%	18.0%	52.8%	88.2%	100%	6.84	2.76
1995	4.8%	16.6%	51.4%	87.0%	100%	7.12	2.77
1996	5.1%	15.2%	52.0%	88.0%	100%	7.52	2.93
1997	3.4%	12.7%	59.4%	92.0%	100%	**7.58**	**2.90**
1998	2.9%	12.4%	59.0%	91.7%	100%	7.67	2.90
1999	3.4%	12.0%	58.7%	91.6%	100%	7.57	2.85
2000	3.3%	11.4%	58.8%	91.5%	100%	7.68	2.88
2001	3.3%	11.4%	58.1%	91.6%	100%	7.67	2.86
2002	4.3%	12.4%	56.8%	91.6%	100%	7.21	2.71

(continued)

Table E.3.2 (continued)

Year	How satisfied are you with your current life as a whole?					Parameters best fit beta distribution	
	Not very satisfied	Fairly satisfied	Satisfied	Very satisfied	Extraordinary satisfied	α	ß
2003	3.6%	12.3%	58.2%	91.3%	100%	7.37	2.78
2004	3.9%	12.0%	58.9%	92.0%	100%	7.52	2.86
2005	4.1%	12.9%	60.7%	92.3%	100%	7.37	2.88
2006	3.4%	12.5%	58.7%	92.2%	100%	***7.64***	***2.90***
2007	3.4%	11.9%	57.8%	92.3%	100%	7.77	2.92
2008	3.4%	11.0%	56.1%	91.6%	100%	7.74	2.84
2009	3.6%	11.8%	54.9%	89.9%	100%	7.13	2.58

Table E.3.3 Cumulative frequencies and parameters beta distribution O-SLL-c-sq-v-5-d, SCP

Year	How satisfied are you with your current life as a whole?					Parameters best fit beta distribution	
	Not very satisfied	Fairly satisfied	Satisfied	Very satisfied	Extraordinary satisfied	α	ß
1974	6.4%	19.6%	62.7%	91.5%	100%	6.85	2.88
1977	6.6%	19.8%	65.2%	91.4%	100%	***6.88***	***2.94***
1989	4.4%	14.9%	47.4%	82.9%	100%	6.13	2.39
1990	4.1%	14.5%	48.7%	84.5%	100%	6.60	2.62
1993	4.0%	12.8%	47.3%	84.7%	100%	***7.22***	***2.82***
1997	3.5%	13.3%	58.8%	92.0%	100%	***7.58***	***2.90***
1999	3.7%	13.1%	60.6%	91.1%	100%	7.35	2.84
2000	4.0%	13.4%	57.4%	91.8%	100%	7.36	2.80

Table E.3.4 Cumulative frequencies and parameters beta distribution O-SLW-c-sq-n-10-a, WVS

	All things considered, how satisfied are you with your life as-a-whole now.....?										Parameters best fit beta distribution	
Year	Dissatisfied	2	3	4	5	6	7	8	9	Satisfied	α	ß
1981	0.2%	1%	2.3%	3.9%	9.8%	17.8%	37.5%	71.6%	85.7%	100%	4.75	1.86
1990	0.5%	1.3%	2.4%	3.6%	8.3%	15.8%	33.1%	70.6%	88.5%	100%	5.23	2.02
1999	0.4%	0.7%	1.2%	1.7%	4.8%	10.4%	30.5%	72.1%	90.6%	100%	7.65	2.75
2006	0.1%	0.4%	0.8%	2.1%	5.4%	13.3%	35.9%	76.2%	90.4%	100%	**7.64**	**2.90**
2008	0.1%	0.3%	0.9%	1.8%	3.5%	7.6%	24.2%	69.1%	91.1%	100%	9.41	3.15
2012	0.2%	0.5%	2%	3.8%	7.1%	16.4%	42.7%	81.7%	96.4%	100%	7.80	3.40

Table E.3.5 Cumulative frequencies and parameters beta distribution O-SLL-c-sq-n-10-a, SCP

	How satisfied are you with the life you currently lead?										Parameters best fit beta distribution	
Year	Completely dissatisfied	2	3	4	5	6	7	8	9	Completely satisfied	α	ß
2004	0.5%	0.7%	1.3%	2.5%	5.4%	14.1%	39.3%	79.3%	93.2%	100%	7.61	2.99
2006	0.4%	0.7%	1.4%	2.1%	5.0%	13.0%	37.4%	77.9%	92.2%	100%	***7.64***	***2.90***
2008	0.2%	0.4%	0.6%	1.6%	3.7%	9.6%	31.9%	74.3%	90.7%	100%	8.36	2.90

Table E.3.6 Cumulative frequencies and parameters beta distribution O-SLW-c-sq-n-11-cd, ESS

	All things considered, how satisfied are you with your life as a whole nowadays?											Parameters best fit beta distribution	
Year	Extremely dissatisfied	1	2	3	4	5	6	7	8	9	Extremely satisfied	α	ß
2002	0.5%	0.9%	1.3%	2.5%	4.5%	8.8%	14.0%	34.0%	73.5%	91.1%	100%	7.19	2.55
2004	0.6%	1.2%	1.7%	2.9%	4.8%	9.1%	16.4%	38.9%	75.5%	92.0%	100%	6.92	2.60
2006	0.4%	0.6%	1.4%	3.1%	5.0%	9.2%	15.3%	38.4%	77.9%	93.6%	100%	***7.64***	***2.90***
2008	0.3%	0.4%	1.1%	2.0%	3.7%	7.1%	12.4%	35.0%	75.5%	93.2%	100%	8.28	2.96
2010	0.3%	0.6%	1.0%	1.8%	3.1%	6.6%	11.7%	30.7%	74.2%	92.7%	100%	8.54	2.93
2012	0.2%	0.4%	0.9%	2.1%	3.3%	6.1%	11.7%	27.0%	66.7%	90.9%	100%	8.07	2.56
2014	0.4%	0.5%	0.8%	1.9%	3.7%	7.3%	14.4%	36.4%	75.8%	93.0%	100%	7.99	2.91

E.4: Cumulative Frequencies and Parameters Beta Distribution Spain (Tables E.4.1, E.4.2, and E.4.3)

Table E.4.1 Cumulative frequencies and parameters beta distribution O-SLL-u-sq-v-4-b, EB

	On the whole how satisfied are you with the life you lead?				Parameters best fit beta distribution	
Year	Not at all satisfied	Not very satisfied	Fairly satisfied	Very satisfied	α	ß
2002	2.4%	16.9%	82.7%	100%	3.78	1.85
2003	1.7%	16.4%	80.5%	100%	3.80	1.77
2004	2.7%	13.3%	69.8%	100%	3.10	1.21
2005	2.2%	14.4%	79.8%	100%	3.85	1.74
2006	1.0%	10.6%	76.4%	100%	4.49	1.78
2007	1.3%	12.6%	78.6%	100%	4.23	1.80
2008	1.8%	15.8%	82.4%	100%	***4.02***	***1.91***
2009	4.3%	22.2%	85.7%	100%	3.26	1.84
2010	5.6%	23.1%	84.1%	100%	2.88	1.63
2011	6.5%	23.9%	84.1%	100%	2.71	1.57
2012	7.4%	29.8%	86.7%	100%	2.57	1.68
2013	8.3%	30.4%	83.9%	100%	2.25	1.44
2014	6.1%	27.7%	82.4%	100%	2.48	1.46
2015	4.0%	22.7%	83.1%	100%	3.06	1.67

Table E.4.2 Cumulative frequencies and parameters beta distribution O-SLW-c-sq-n-10-a, WVS

	All things considered, how satisfied are you with your life as-a-whole now.....?										Parameters best fit beta distribution	
Year	Dissatisfied	2	3	4	5	6	7	8	9	Satisfied	α	ß
1981	1.3%	2.9%	7.2%	15.0%	28.5%	43.2%	65.6%	84.8%	91.5%	100%	2.90	1.86
1990	1.1%	2.1%	4.6%	7.7%	20.0%	33.3%	53.2%	76.5%	87.8%	100%	3.20	1.63
1995	1.2%	2.2%	6.0%	11.4%	29.6%	45.5%	74.5%	76.7%	91.9%	100%	2.97	1.88
1999	1.4%	2.7%	5.7%	9.7%	20.7%	33.0%	54.0%	75.9%	87.6%	100%	2.89	1.51
2000	0.8%	1.5%	3.9%	6.7%	20.6%	36.3%	60.3%	80.9%	89.8%	100%	3.64	1.97
2007	0.3%	0.5%	1.8%	3.9%	10.9%	24.7%	51.7%	79.9%	94.1%	100%	5.99	2.81
2008	0.8%	1.5%	4.2%	7.5%	15.4%	25.2%	45.5%	77.5%	90.8%	100%	**4.02**	**1.91**
2011	0.9%	1.8%	4.2%	8.9%	22.7%	37.9%	63.5%	86.7%	94.1%	100%	4.07	2.42

Table E.4.3 Cumulative frequencies and parameters beta distribution O-SLW-c-sq-n-11-cd, ESS

	All things considered, how satisfied are you with your life as a whole nowadays?										Parameters best fit beta distribution	
Year	Extremely dissatisfied	ß	2	3	4	5	6	7	8	9	Extremely satisfied	α	ß
2002	0.4%	1%	2.4%	4.9%	8.1%	18.6%	31.8%	55.6%	80%	89%	100%	3.56	1.87
2004	0.9%	1.3%	2.7%	4.9%	8.4%	18.4%	29.9%	51.8%	78.9%	89.6%	100%	3.53	1.81
2006	0.5%	1.1%	2.2%	3.6%	5.4%	13%	22.9%	44.1%	74.2%	88.9%	100%	4.07	1.82
2008	0.3%	0.6%	1.5%	3.8%	7.6%	16.3%	25.6%	46.4%	76.8%	90.3%	100%	***4.02***	***1.91***
2010	0.7%	1%	1.4%	3.1%	6.1%	14.8%	25.1%	48%	78.8%	91.1%	100%	4.31	2.07
2012	2.4%	3.2%	5.5%	9.3%	13.3%	24.4%	35.3%	53%	75.6%	86.9%	100%	2.47	1.36
2014	0.4%	0.5%	0.8%	1.9%	3.7%	7.3%	14.4%	36.4%	75.8%	93.0%	100%	7.99	2.91

Glossary

Anchor point Response option at the beginning or the end of a discrete scale.

Beta distribution Continuous distribution on a two-sided bounded continuum with shape parameters α and β.

Continuum approach A method to estimate a population mean and standard deviation of the continuous cumulative distribution function that best fits the points on a common, bounded continuum at which response options for a given response scale transit from one to another combined with the frequency distribution of the primary response scale.

Extreme The boundary of the continuum within which the range of values of a continuous distribution falls.

Happiness scale interval study Study to look at survey questions on happiness using verbal response options with the intent to determine consistently what degrees of happiness are denoted by the labels used for these options when the questions are asked in different languages and different subpopulations are addressed.

(In)comparability problem The incomparability of survey results due to differences in response scales used.

Item A survey question and its corresponding response options.

Linear stretch method Transformation method by which a discrete primary scale is transformed in such a way that the rank of the 'lowest' response option is always projected onto 0 and the 'highest' onto the highest value of the range, and all the intermediate options are given equally spaced numbers in between the two points.

Numerical scale Response scale with a discrete number of response options, with only the anchor points labeled verbally and all other response options labeled with a number.

Rank method Method according to which the sample mean is calculated as the weighted average of the ranks of the response options using the relative frequencies as weights.

Rating scale Discrete response scale to rate the response to a survey question.

T. de Jonge et al., *Diversity in Survey Questions on the Same Topic*, Social Indicators Research Series 68, DOI 10.1007/978-3-319-53261-5

Reference boundary Boundary between two response options of a discrete primary response scale derived from a reference distribution for the frequency distribution in the same year as the year on which the reference distribution is based.

Reference distribution Continuous cumulative distribution based on an appropriate primary scale and frequency distribution in a given year to be used as a reference to derive reference boundaries for the response options of a discrete primary scale given the frequency distribution for this primary scale in the same year as the year on which the reference distribution is based.

Reference distribution method Method according to which the boundaries between the response options of a primary scale are derived from a reference distribution given the frequency distribution for this primary scale is in the same year as the year on which the reference distribution is based, and for samples from the same population.

Scale interval method Method according to which judges assess the points on a common, bounded continuum in which verbal response options for a given response scale transit from one to another. A population mean and standard deviation are estimated using the Continuum Approach.

Scale interval recorder Web-based instrument to be used for the assessment of the points on a common, bounded continuum at which verbal response options for a given response scale transit from one option to another.

Scale transformation Transformation of the response options of a primary scale into numerical secondary ratings, usually on a common range.

Semantic judgment of fixed word value method Method according to which fixed values are assigned to the labels of verbal response options, based on the rating by experts of a series of qualifications that can be given to verbal response options on a common numerical scale. The sample mean is calculated using the Weighted Average Approach.

Translation bias Poor comparability of data due to the translation phenomenon where adverbs used in a label of a response options are not necessarily translated to a synonymous adverb in the translation language, thus causing errors of nuancing, for example by judges judging survey items.

Verbal scale Response scale with a discrete number of response options labeled with descriptive text.

Weighted average approach Method according to which the sample mean for a survey item is calculated as the weighted average of the values assigned to the response options of a discrete scale using the relative frequencies as weights. Generalization of the Rank Method, as it is not required that the numbers assigned to the response options are equal to the ranks of these response options to calculate a sample mean.

World database of happiness Archive of research findings on subjective enjoyment of one's life as a whole. The procedure to estimate the population mean and standard deviation presented in this book were developed in the context of this project (go to: http://worlddatabaseofhappiness.eur.nl/).

MIX
Papier aus verantwortungsvollen Quellen
Paper from responsible sources
FSC® C105338

If you have any concerns about our products,
you can contact us on
ProductSafety@springernature.com

In case Publisher is established outside the EU,
the EU authorized representative is:
Springer Nature Customer Service Center GmbH
Europaplatz 3, 69115 Heidelberg, Germany

Printed by Libri Plureos GmbH
in Hamburg, Germany